THE PARAMEDIC REVIEW MANUAL

Jonathan F. Politis, BA, REMT-P
Judith A. Cremeens, RN, MA Ed, REMT-P
Patricia L. Tritt, RN, BS

W.B. SAUNDERS COMPANY
A Division of Harcourt Brace & Company

W.B. SAUNDERS COMPANY
A Division of
Harcourt Brace & Company

The Curtis Center
Independence Square West
Philadelphia, Pennsylvania 19106

ISBN 0-7216-5041-4

In the writing of this review manual, the contributing authors, editors, and publisher have made every attempt to follow current practices in prehospital emergency care. Suggested drug selections and dosages conform to current protocols at the time of publication. Treatment techniques are reviewed with equal concern for the most uniformly accepted protocols and procedures. It is the responsibility of the reader to conform to local standards and to be aware of new research conclusions, technological advancements, and government regulations that dictate changes which may alter suggested drug therapies or treatment protocols.

Contributing Authors

Judith A. Cremeens, RN, MA Ed, REMT-P
Ass't. Professor of Emergency Medical Care
Eastern Kentucky University
Richmond, KY

Jonathan F. Politis, BA, REMT-P
Director, Emergency Medical Services
Town of Colonie
Newtonville, NY

Patricia L. Tritt, RN, BS
Director of Prehospital Services
Swedish Medical Center
Englewood, CO

Manuscript Reviewers

Todd J. Brekken, MS, NREMT-P
Ass't Professor, Emergency Medical Care Program
Eastern Kentucky University
Richmond, KY

Donna J. Duell, RN, MS
Director, Department of Nursing
Cabrillo College
Soquel, CA

Mark Lockhart, NEMT-P
Director, Department of Paramedic Education
St. John's Mercy Medical Center
St. Louis, MO
President (1991-1992) National Association Emergency Medical Technicians

Donald J. Ptacnik, EMT
EMS Consulting
Bend, OR

Sandra Rehmar, RN, MS, MICN, EMT-P
Program Coordinator
Stanford Prehospital Care Program
Palo Alto, CA

Preface

The purpose of this review manual is to develop your confidence to pass the certification examination for EMT-Paramedic. If you are currently certified, this book will provide you with an effective review aid for your refresher and/or recertification requirements.

The Paramedic Review Manual consists of multiple-choice questions accompanied by answers and rationale. The questions are organized into chapters that parallel the US DOT EMT-Paramedic training modules. You will be able to conduct a thorough analysis of your strengths and weaknesses by tabulating your results on each of the main topics covered by the questions. Reading the rationale accompanying the answers will provide you with an additional learning experience.

The material in the first chapter, "Developing Your Test-Taking Skills," will explain the examination's overall purpose and format. In addition, you will find valuable suggestions on review strategies and test-taking techniques.

The contributing authors and manuscript reviewers have extensive backgrounds in EMT-Paramedic education. Their questions will test your knowledge and understanding of material covered in the EMT-Paramedic training programs.

This review manual can also serve you on a continuing basis. These questions will help you to remain familiar with data that may have become somewhat "fuzzy" through lack of use.

The true test, of course, comes when you are called upon in the field to make assessments and take actions under emergency conditions. A broad knowledge base and confidence in your own ability to recall and apply that knowledge are key factors for success. Periodic study and review will help you in your continuing pursuit of excellence in emergency care.

Jonathan F. Politis   Judith A. Cremeens   Patricia L. Tritt

Contents

1 Developing Your Test-Taking Skills

Introduction

Over the years, EMT-Paramedic testing in the United States has undergone significant changes in an effort to achieve standardization and maintain high standards. Individual states administer standardized examinations to: (1) ensure that only qualified and competent individuals are certified for EMS positions, (2) conform more closely to national standards, and (3) promote career mobility. As a candidate for EMT-Paramedic certification, you should be aware of these trends and use them to your advantage while preparing for your State or National Registry examination.

Knowing how to take tests effectively involves techniques and strategies that are developed and enhanced through practice. The ability to prepare for and then actually take a crucial test can be nearly as important as mastering the basic knowledge.

This chapter provides you with a perspective on the design and structure typical of certification examinations. Other topics covered include study guidelines, test-taking strategies, and helpful hints for use during the actual exam.

Test Blueprint

Just as an architect's blueprint specifies the overall structure and components of a building, certification examinations also follow a general design. The test blueprint specifies the topics to be covered and the number of questions to be included in each section or subsection. State and National Registry written examinations for EMT-P are multiple-choice tests. They have minimum overall scores and, in some cases, minimum subtest scores as well. The rationale behind the subtest structure is to ensure that certification candidates are knowledgeable in all major phases of prehospital advanced life support.

Test Format

A multiple-choice test item consists of a problem and several alternative answers. The problem, called the **stem**, may be stated as a direct question or an incomplete statement. Four alternatives follow the stem. You are expected to read the stem and alternatives and to select the correct, or most correct, alternative. The correct alternative is the answer, while the remaining alternatives are called **distractors**.

Most test items are generated from specific knowledge objectives contained in your State or National curriculum. The objectives of your training program should have been similar, if not identical, to the ones emphasized on your EMT-P exam. The specific test items will require four different thought processes:

- Recognition—your ability to recognize or identify something you have already learned (e.g., a medical definition).
- Recall—your ability to supply the answer based on your knowledge of the topic (e.g., steps in starting an IV).
- Problem solving—your ability to apply facts and principles to a given situation (e.g., figuring drug dosages or interpreting rhythms).
- Decision making—your ability to demonstrate critical thinking (e.g., presented with multiple data on a patient's condition and mechanism of injury, you are asked to make a treatment decision).

As mentioned previously, you will have to select the correct, or most correct, answer. This may be a source of frustration since a multiple-choice test requiring a "most correct" selection tends to be more difficult than an exam asking you to select only the correct answer. You will be forced to discriminate among several alternatives, all of which may appear to be correct. In some cases, there may be partially correct answers in more than one alternative, but the correct answer will be the **most correct** alternative.

Types of Test Questions

You will encounter two basic types of multiple-choice test questions, or items, on your EMT-P examination: simple and compound. The **simple** multiple-choice item is the most commonly used question form. Generally, it tests recall of factual and procedural material. Questions 1 and 2 are examples of the simple item.

Example Question

1. Which area of the nervous system is responsible for the functions of heart rate, respiration, and blood pressure?

   A. Cerebral cortex.
   B. Medulla.
   C. Cerebellum.
   D. Thalamus.

   The correct answer is (B). The medulla controls a variety of cardiorespiratory functions. Therefore, damage to the medulla can result in cardiopulmonary arrest.

Example Question

2. Proper handling of an amputated body part includes which of the following?

   A. Applying a tourniquet to the amputated part.
   B. Immersing the part in .045 normal saline solution.
   C. Wrapping the part in a dry, sterile dressing and freezing.
   D. Wrapping the part in a moist, sterile dressing and placing it in a plastic bag.

   The correct answer is (D). It is important to prevent the amputated part from drying out or from coming in contact with external debris.

   The **compound** multiple-choice item provides you with a combination of possible alternatives from which you must select the most correct combination. These items usually involve critical thinking and require you to apply a combination of recognition, recall, and problem-solving to a specific situation. Questions 3 and 4 are examples of the compound item.

Example Question

3. A 14-year-old girl fell approximately 13 feet from a tree house to the ground. She is complaining of pain in her left leg. Which of the following should be performed while examining her for possible injuries to her leg?

   (1) Palpate the area of injury.
   (2) Palpate for arterial flow to the extremity.
   (3) Bend the leg gently to elicit grating or crepitus.
   (4) Gently touch the left foot with a sharp object to elicit neural response.

   A. 1, 2.
   B. 2, 4.
   C. 1, 2, 4.
   D. 1, 2, 3, 4.

   The correct answer is (D). Initial palpation of the injured area is important to determine if there are associated injuries and to assess adequate blood flow. Gentle manipulation helps identify the presence of a long-bone fracture. Nerve integrity is evaluated by using a sharp object.

Example Question

4. You are called to the home of a 28-year-old obese female in her third trimester of pregnancy. She complains of headaches, appears edematous, is hyperactive, and is frightened. Her vital signs are pulse 105, respirations 22, and BP 280/110. As you complete your assessment, the patient experiences a clonic-tonic seizure. Which of the following would be included in the management of this patient?

   (1) Oxygen, 6 L/cannula.
   (2) Magnesium sulfate 1–2 gm in 50 cc, D_5W, TKO.
   (3) IV D_5W, TKO.
   (4) Lasix 40 mg IV.
   (5) Fluid challenge of 20 cc/kg, NS or LR.

A. 1, 3.
B. 1, 2, 3.
C. 1, 2, 3, 4.
D. 1, 2, 4, 5.

The correct answer is (B). The history is suggestive of eclampsia. Appropriate management includes oxygen, magnesium sulfate, and an IV of D_5W, TKO. Magnesium sulfate is the drug of choice to treat eclamptic seizures. However, if it is not stocked in the field, Valium may be ordered. Despite the edema, Lasix is not indicated in the field. The patient is hypertensive and a fluid challenge is contraindicated.

Reviewing for the Exam

Many candidates for EMT-P certification are unable to take the exam immediately upon the conclusion of their training program. Quarterly or even biannual examinations are common in many states. The delay before testing, combined with long travel and overnight lodging in an unfamiliar city, can create additional test anxiety. To combat such stresses, it is important that you develop a specific review plan to prepare for your State or National Registry examination.

Several weeks before your test date, you should meet with your instructor or several other candidates for a study session. Review the overall scope of the course. Organize your pertinent notes, handouts, tests, and quizzes. Become familiar with the test blueprint and reevaluate your personal strengths and weaknesses regarding the material for which you will be held responsible.

A most effective way of determining your strengths and weaknesses is to answer the questions in this book and evaluate your results. These practice questions will expose you to a wide variety of topics and writing styles. State or National Registry exams may phrase questions quite differently from your instructor.

Practice questions can increase your speed in completing the examination. This is important because most exams are timed to allow one minute per question (e.g., for a 150-item exam, you are usually allowed 2 1/2 hours). This can pose a problem if you read slowly or ponder too long over a compound multiple-choice item. Practice testing under time constraints.

As you score your results on each test, read the entire rationale accompanying the answers. If this material is unclear or contradicts other information you have learned, consult your textbooks or contact your instructor for clarification.

Once you have sorted out your strong areas from your weaker ones, you know what to emphasize during your study sessions. It is important that you allocate your study time with similar emphasis to the structure of the exam. It is a mistake to study only topics that you like (e.g., Cardiology) to the exclusion of other seemingly less important areas (e.g., OB/GYN, Pediatrics/Neonatal). The subjects you like are probably those that you know best and where your confidence level is high. Focus on topics whose questions you missed in this book. Also, relate your study time to the relative importance of these subjects on the examination.

Plan your daily study time. Do not schedule study time during portions of the day when you are the most tired or preoccupied with the day's activities. Arrange to study when you are mentally alert and fresh. In scheduling your time, be realistic. You should review all important material. Spend extra time on material that gives you the most trouble. Ask yourself what types of questions and thought processes need the most review. Then you can use your class notes, handouts, and textbooks most efficiently.

Develop flash cards or note cards as a study aid. You will be surprised at how much information, particularly recall and recognition material, you can get on a 3 X 5 card. Medical terms, abbreviations, short definitions, procedures, drug dosages, indications/contraindications, and ECG characteristics are easily transported in your pocket or purse. Outside of your planned study time, there are usually blocks of free minutes available throughout your day. Use these opportunities to drill yourself.

24-Hour Countdown

The following suggestions apply to your activities during the time period just prior to your exam.

1. Get a normal night's rest. Being rested and fresh will add more points to your score than any last-minute cramming.

2. If you have to travel a long distance to the examination site, (e.g., two hours or greater) you will probably be more relaxed for the exam if you travel the day before and spend the preceding night in a motel.

3. Avoid partying, or using stimulants or depressants, prior to the exam. There will be sufficient time to celebrate after the test.

4. A moderate breakfast should help keep you from becoming fatigued during the exam. Avoid too much caffeine as it may cause you to be jittery.

5. Review rules or guidelines sent to you by your State or the National Registry. Will you need picture ID? Pencils? Calipers? Calculator? Watch?

Test-Taking Strategies

Some EMT-P candidates fail the certification examination for reasons other than lack of knowledge. The following should assist you at the examination site and will help you to attain the best possible score. As you enter the test site, you should:

1. Select a seat away from friends. Also, avoid drafts, darkened areas, windows, and other potential distractions.

2. If you are left-handed but the desks are designed for right-handed individuals, ask if a second desk is available to gain a more comfortable writing position.

3. Listen to the test proctor's instructions. How long is the exam? Will the time remaining be periodically announced? Are calculators or calipers allowed? What is the policy regarding stretch breaks or smoking?

4. Determine how the examination is scored. Do guesses count against you? If not, making a guess is better than leaving an answer blank. If the exam is computer scored, do you understand the layout of the score sheet?

During the test itself, you can follow certain strategies to enhance your results. These include:

1. Do not read extra meaning into the question. If necessary, rephrase the question in your own words so that it is clear in your mind. Ask yourself "What is the question asking?" and look for key words or phrases.

2. Understand the stem completely before considering the alternatives. Is it asking for the right or wrong response? Recognize stems with specific qualifiers such as *best*, *least*, or *most*. Beware of alternatives that contain specific qualifiers like *always* or *never*.

3. Look for similarities in two or three of the choices, remembering that the purpose of distractors is to divert you from the answer and that you must choose the most correct answer.

4. After choosing what you feel is the correct answer, go back to the stem and make sure your choice answers the question. Remember, an alternative may be correct as it stands by itself, but incorrect in terms of what the question is asking.

5. If you have no clue concerning the correct answer, often the most comprehensive alternative is correct. This is particularly true of similar alternatives, with one more detailed than the others.

6. Be cautious about changing your mind after answering a question. Usually, your initial "hunch" is valid. Let your intuition work in your favor. If a subsequent question sheds new information and causes you to recognize your previous mistake, then go back and change the answer.

7. Occasionally an answer to one question is accidentally given away in a following question.

8. Periodically check your watch to make sure you are progressing through the test in reasonable time. It is better to leave time-consuming questions unanswered to the end and be able to finish the entire exam than to risk not finishing or frustrating yourself early in the exam.

9. If you are using a computer answer sheet, periodically check that you are answering in the correct order. Being just one place off will make all following answers incorrect. If you skip a question, be sure to skip the appropriate answer.

10. Avoid unnecessary erasures or stray marks. Missing answers and multiple answers will be scored as incorrect.

11. When confronted with a compound multiple-choice question, read the stem and consider points that are incorrect before proceeding to the alternatives. It is usually easier to recognize incorrect information than to discriminate among correct items. Review the listed items and identify those which are incorrect. Look at the distractors and eliminate those which contain the wrong items. If two or more selections remain, compare them to

determine similarities and differences. Continued elimination is generally possible by determining what is the same and what is different. This process will spare time as well as prevent inadvertent errors due to confusion as you attempt to remember each detail about the subject.

12. Be aware of questions that ask you to select an incorrect response, the *"except"* questions. Generally, "except" will appear at the end of a stem and will be italicized, underlined, or bold-faced to alert you. Similarly, "not true" is usually highlighted. This may not be true in all cases. Therefore, you must be alert to this possibility when reading the stem and make sure that all responses are read. When you think there is more than one correct response, review the stem to assure it is not an "except" question. As you read the responses, ask yourself, "What is not true about . . . ?" This will serve as a constant reminder about what you are looking for in the answer.

13. Preventing panic while taking a timed examination is essential to improving your results. This can be accomplished by not expending inordinate amounts of time on questions which you cannot initially answer with confidence. As you progress from question to question, you may encounter some which do not appear familiar or which you cannot provide an immediate, confident response. In these cases, simply skip it and go on to the next until you have made it through all of the questions. Then go back and answer those which you left blank. This process may require two, three, or more rounds of going back before you have answered all of the questions. You have, however, removed the pressure of completing the examination within a specified time frame as well as obtained credit for questions answered correctly which may have gone unanswered because insufficient time remained after struggling over a few questions. Removing the pressure will also allow you to read unanswered questions more closely which usually makes the correct answer more apparent. Remember to periodically check the answer sheet and question numbers to make sure you are marking the correct area for each question.

14. When you have completed the examination, review your answer sheet. Count the number of marks to assure the same number of responses as questions. This will prevent double responses for one question as well as provide you with an opportunity to ensure all questions have been answered.

In summary, these strategies are guidelines, not absolutes. Always use your own judgment, knowledge, and experience. These assets will serve you in passing EMT-P certification exams. You have the background, education, and knowledge. Be confident that you will pass and, in fact, you will.

2

Prehospital Environment

Roles, Responsibilities, and EMS Systems

1. As a newly graduated paramedic, you have been assigned to the dispatch center for your orientation. When receiving a call, what is the most important information to obtain before possibly losing contact with a hysterical caller?

   A. Nature of the event.
   B. Potential scene hazards.
   C. Call-back number.
   D. Cross street names.

2. You have responded to an accident involving three vehicles (one of which has been on fire), and there are six patients. You direct your EMT partner to begin assessment of the least critical patients while you begin advanced life support intervention on a critically burned 33-year-old female. What would be a justifiable basis for your direction to your Basic EMT partner?

   A. You have confidence in the skill level of the Basic EMT.
   B. You have been authorized to do so by the Medical Director.
   C. The duties are commensurate with the Basic EMT abilities.
   D. There are multiple casualties.

3. You are a firefighter/paramedic on the scene of a multivictim accident. With you are police, a fire engine crew, and a BLS-trained ambulance crew. You rapidly establish contact with your hospital base station. Who is ultimately responsible for patient care?

   A. The base station physician.
   B. You, the paramedic.
   C. The highest-ranking fire officer.
   D. The nurse on the radio.

4. Upon completion of your paramedic course, you participate in a testing process designed by the state agency to find out if you meet certain predetermined qualifications. If you are successful in this process, you will be granted:

   A. Licensure.
   B. Certification.
   C. Credentials.
   D. Legal affirmation.

5. What is your best protection against the threat of being named as a defendant in a negligence case?

   A. Malpractice insurance.
   B. Never taking undue risks.
   C. High standard of training.
   D. There is nothing you can do.

6. Your base station has just given you an order for 50 mg of lidocaine IV push for a patient experiencing frequent PVCs. After injecting the medication, you discover it was a 100-mg preload instead of 50 mg. You should:

   A. Forget about it; the extra 50 mg will not be injurious.
   B. Immediately report the error to the base station.
   C. Say nothing. The base station will probably order another 50 mg before you get there anyway, and it will even out.
   D. Report it to the base station or receiving hospital after the run is over, so you can restock your supplies.

7. Both the 1980 and 1985 revised KKK-A-1822 specifications were developed to improve ambulance:

   (1) Design.
   (2) Personnel.
   (3) Function.
   (4) Reliability.
   (5) Safety.

   A. 1, 2, 4.
   B. 1, 3, 5.
   C. 2, 4, 5.
   D. 3, 4, 5.

8. While you are rendering care to a victim of an automobile accident, a man approaches you. He informs you that he is a family practice physician and wants to help the patient. This situation is best managed by:

   A. Contacting Medical Control on the radio and allowing him to speak with the base hospital physician.
   B. Thanking him for his interest and asking politely that he leave the scene.

C. Asking for verification of licensure and yielding to his expertise upon receipt of such verification.
D. Informing him that only the EMS Medical Director can give EMS personnel orders.

9. When you are unable to contact the base physician by radio, advanced-level patient care is possible with standard operating procedures or established protocols that have been developed by the Medical Director to provide:

A. Off-line Medical Control.
B. On-line Medical Control.
C. Direct Medical Control.
D. Quality assurance.

10. You are preparing to transport a stable patient to your base station hospital when he requests to be taken to another hospital in the community. He states that his private physician is on staff at the facility and will be waiting for him. Your partner begins to explain the problems he has had with that particular facility and why the patient would receive better treatment at the base hospital. Your partner's behavior is:

A. Illegal.
B. In the best interest of the patient.
C. Unethical.
D. Justifiable when you hear the reasons.

11. You have been asked to attend a meeting to discuss ordering new ambulances. During the meeting there is debate about buying Type I or Type III units. What is the major difference between these two designs?

A. Type I has a raised roof; Type III does not.
B. Type III has a passageway between the driver's and patient's compartments; Type I does not.
C. Type I is a standard van construction; Type III is modular.
D. Type III meets all standards entitling it to bear the "Star of Life" symbol; Type I must be customized by the service to meet these standards.

Medical/Legal Issues

12. You are working in a state that has an established Good Samaritan law. As a certified paramedic, you are afforded what protection under this legislation?

    A. Probable prevention of litigation after introducing the Good Samaritan law as the basis of intervention.
    B. Complete ability to perform your advanced life support skills without fear of lawsuits.
    C. Absolute legal immunity only when functioning as an unpaid, volunteer paramedic.
    D. Possible protection from ultimate liability if the Good Samaritan law is applicable as a defense.

13. The mother of a pregnant 14-year-old patient insists that you transport her daughter to the hospital for a psychiatric evaluation because the daughter has recently been depressed. You make contact with the patient, but she refuses care and transport. What is the best action in this situation?

    A. Transport only; based on valid consent from parents.
    B. Nontransport; based on obvious domestic dispute.
    C. Nontransport; based on legal refusal from the patient.
    D. Treat and transport; based on implied consent.

14. In order to obtain a legal judgment citing negligence, the plaintiff must prove all of the following *except*:

    A. Treatment without consent.
    B. Proximate cause.
    C. Breach of duty.
    D. Damages.

15. You have been named in a lawsuit charging negligence in the care of a 17-year-old female involved in a motorcycle accident. The suit claims permanent disability and disfigurement from improper management of a femur fracture. The suit contends that your management caused a closed midshaft fracture to become an open fracture. Four years after the accident, your best legal protection is afforded by:

A. Eyewitness testimony from your EMT partner confirming appropriate action was taken to stabilize the fracture.
B. A copy of the ambulance call sheet submitted as part of the hospital records.
C. An audio cassette tape of your voice communicating that a traction splint was applied to a closed femur fracture.
D. Your testimony, under oath, that a traction splint was applied prior to moving the patient.

16. Dispatch assigns your unit to "a person down." On arrival, you find an unresponsive male who has, according to bystanders, experienced a generalized motor seizure. As you begin the primary assessment, the patient begins to seize again. Intervention is possible by virtue of:

A. Implied consent.
B. Expressed consent.
C. Involuntary consent.
D. Voluntary consent—special circumstances.

17. A 57-year-old patient, whose chief complaint is chest pain, has called you to his home. You identify yourself as a paramedic, and he consents to your examination and treatment. He is showing classic signs and symptoms of acute MI with pain that seems severe, and he pleads with you to do something for the pain. The monitor is showing 10–16 PVCs per minute. This patient has no previous history of heart problems. You have contacted your base station and have just brought out the catheter to start the IV. The patient sees it and frantically orders you to stop, saying, "I don't care what happens, you're not sticking that needle into me!" Despite every effort from you and your partner to obtain consent for this procedure, the patient will not allow it. What should you do now?

A. Have him arrested as a danger to himself, and then begin treatment.
B. Inform him that he cannot withdraw consent once he has given it, and proceed to treat.
C. Proceed to treat him regardless of his withdrawal of consent, because his life is in danger.
D. Inform him of the possible consequences of his refusal of the procedure, and obtain his signature on a release form.

18. In most cases, charges of negligence stem from an act of:

    A. Omission.
    B. Commission.
    C. Authority.
    D. Disregard for the family.

19. You are on a nonemergency call to the home of Thelma Wilson, who is 80 years old. You are informed by Medical Control that she is to be transported to a local hospital for admission by her physician, who believes Thelma has suffered a stroke. Thelma refuses to go and claims her son and family are after her money. She wanders off, calling for her cat. Who can authorize you to transport Thelma against her will?

    A. Her son.
    B. Her physician.
    C. The court.
    D. Medical Control.

20. You have just placed a nursing home patient onto a stretcher in the Emergency Department when dispatch informs all units to respond to a multi-vehicle accident on the interstate highway. You direct your crew to make the cot en route and proceed directly to the accident scene. Which statement best describes your action in this situation?

    A. Justifiable based on a possible mass-casualty situation.
    B. Abandonment if report was not given on the patient.
    C. Negligent only if the dispatch report is incorrect.
    D. Appropriate because the nursing home-to-hospital interfacility transfer is not an emergency situation.

21. You have just treated a well-known public official for a drug overdose. As you leave the Emergency Department, you find yourself surrounded by members of the press, all of whom are urgently questioning you about your patient. You should:

    A. Deny that you cared for this patient or that you know about him.
    B. Tell them who it was, what you saw, and what you did.
    C. Admit to caring for the patient, but nothing more.
    D. Tactfully tell them they will have to talk to a representative from the hospital.

22. Your patient is a 5-year-old female who has taken a bad fall down stairs. The mother says that you can treat her, but the father tells you to leave, that he'll take care of "his own kid." Which of the following statements is *not* true for this situation?

    A. Permission from both parents is required before treating the child.
    B. Permission from only one parent is required before treating the child.
    C. If the parents are divorced, the parent with physical custody has the right of consent.
    D. If both parents deny consent to treat, you cannot "just go ahead and treat," even if you feel the child is seriously ill or injured.

23. You have treated and transported a 4-year-old patient who has a bruised elbow and edematous left arm from an injury received three days prior. When asked about the delay, the parents state they just returned from vacation. They say the child was staying at his grandparents' house. The parents also mention that the child has not been seen by a physician since he was 6 months old. After delivery to the Emergency Department, you should:

    A. Confide your concerns to the physician.
    B. Document your suspicions on the ambulance report form.
    C. Complete and file a form to report suspected child abuse or neglect.
    D. Say nothing to prejudice hospital personnel, because they will take the appropriate action.

24. Your patient is a 47-year-old male who is experiencing chest pain and shortness of breath. After completing the physical examination, you prepare to start an IV of 5% DW. At this time, the patient informs you to take him directly to the hospital without the IV. What potential legal risk would you incur by completing the IV as ordered in your protocol?

    A. Negligence.
    B. Battery.
    C. Malfeasance.
    D. Assault.

25. After completing an ambulance report form, you note a documentation error. Because the form is pressure sensitive to produce additional copies, how could you correct your error?

A. Draw a single line through it and initial the line.
B. Use a correcting liquid on all copies and write the correction on the whitened area.
C. Void the entire form, retrieve all copies, and write a new one.
D. Blacken the error with as many lines as necessary, star the area, and make the correction.

26. As you are preparing to transport a cardiac patient to the hospital, the family informs you the attending physician and patient previously agreed to limited intervention if arrest occurs. They state that if the patient's heart stops, he is to receive only cardiac medication. They are explicit about no "chest compressions, tubes, or shocks." What should you do if the patient arrests en route?

A. Implement advanced cardiopulmonary arrest management.
B. Abide by their wishes and administer medications only.
C. Contact Medical Control before doing anything.
D. Administer basic life support as minimal care.

27. Dispatch notifies you that a patient is experiencing third trimester vaginal hemorrhage. As your unit approaches the subdivision, you realize this location is not in your response area. You would:

A. Notify dispatch and return to service.
B. Have dispatch contact the area's EMS agency and leave.
C. Contact the hospital to notify the appropriate provider.
D. Respond to the scene and manage the case accordingly.

28. A hospice nurse calls EMS because a patient has a high fever associated with nausea and vomiting. Once you arrive, the nurse tells you the patient has terminal cancer and shows you the doctor's DNR order. The patient is hypotensive and vomiting large amounts of clear emesis. You would transport:

A. And provide emotional support.
B. To the hospital without intervention.
C. And ignore the DNR order in the case of cardiac arrest.
D. With an established IV line for fluid replacement.

29. A 68-year-old male is in cardiopulmonary arrest. Upon your arrival, the family presents the patient's Living Will. What should you do in this situation?

A. Continue with resuscitative efforts as implied consent.
B. Have the family sign a refusal form and leave.
C. Honor the document and notify the coroner or medical examiner's office.
D. Contact Medical Control as soon as possible after securing the airway and establishing an IV access.

EMS Communications

30. Select the correct sequence for communicating the following information:

   (1) Pulse 116 and regular; respirations 26 and shallow; blood pressure 150/96.
   (2) NKA.
   (3) Experiencing RUQ pain.
   (4) 57-year-old female.

   A. 4, 1, 3, 2.
   B. 4, 3, 2, 1.
   C. 1, 4, 3, 2.
   D. 3, 1, 4, 2.

31. All of the following are functions of the Federal Communications Commission (FCC) *except*:

   A. Issuing frequency and license regulations.
   B. Conducting spot checks of base stations and their records.
   C. Monitoring assigned radio frequencies.
   D. Providing funds for biotelemetry communications.

32. During your orientation to an EMS unit, the paramedic supervisor explains that the Emergency Medical Service system uses a duplex communication system. You realize that from the field you are able to transmit:

   A. Voice and telemetry, simultaneously, on one frequency.
   B. Voice or telemetry, in only one mode at a time, using one frequency.
   C. Voice and telemetry, simultaneously, on separate frequencies.
   D. Voice or telemetry, in either mode, using two frequencies.

33. You are assessing a patient who complains of chest pain. After applying the ECG electrodes, you obtain the following tracing:

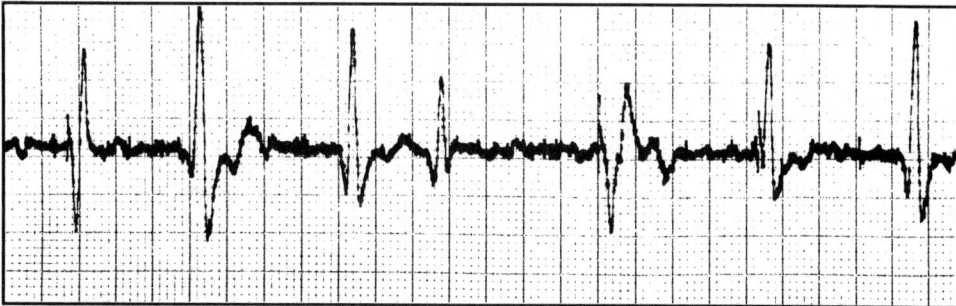

You recognize the problem as:

A. Faulty electrode interface.
B. Monitor battery failure.
C. Muscle tremor artifact.
D. Sixty-cycle interference.

34. As your partner continues the care for a patient who was involved in a one-car accident, you prepare to contact the base station. When your first attempt is unsuccessful, you recognize the need to extend the mobile unit's transmission range. This requires the use of which of the following?

A. Repeater.
B. Encoder.
C. Decoder.
D. Acoustic coupler.

35. Which of the following statements best describes a remote console?

A. Resembles a telephone dial that causes pulsed tones to be sent out over the air when dialed.
B. Receives a signal on one frequency and retransmits that signal on another frequency.
C. Receives only properly coded messages.
D. Is a control console connected to the base station by telephone lines.

36. Select the essential components of an emergency communications system:

    (1) Emergency telephone notification system.
    (2) Dispatch of emergency personnel.
    (3) Communication between dispatcher and vehicles.
    (4) Communication between physicians and paramedics.
    (5) Interhospital communications.

    A. 1, 2, 3.
    B. 1, 2, 3, 4.
    C. 1, 2, 3, 4, 5.
    D. 2, 3, 4, 5.

37. All of the following factors will decrease the range of a mobile transmitter/receiver *except*:

    A. Dense foliage.
    B. Mountainous terrain.
    C. Water.
    D. Urban areas.

38. Which of the following maximizes the range for low-power mobile or portable transmitter/receiver units?

    A. Satellite receivers.
    B. Encoders.
    C. Decoders.
    D. Remote consoles.

39. The dispatcher must gather data from the caller requesting help. The data should include all of the following *except*:

    A. Nature of the call.
    B. Call-back number.
    C. Caller's location.
    D. Past medical history.

40. Which of the following guidelines is most appropriate when speaking into the radio?

    A. Speak in a monotone.
    B. Use codes in all situations.

C. Speak 2 to 3 inches from the microphone.

D. Voice activate the system prior to using the frequency.

41. Which of the following best protects the patient's right of privacy during field-to-base communications?

A. Avoid using the patient's name.

B. Communicate with ten-codes.

C. Employ echo procedure for orders.

D. Utilize the telephone.

Rescue/Major Incident Response

42. You are preparing to extricate the driver of an automobile involved in an accident. The patient appears stable. Which of the following adjuncts for initial spinal immobilization is most appropriate if a spinal injury is suspected?

A. CID.

B. KED.

C. Long wooden backboard.

D. Orthopedic or scoop stretcher.

43. A luxury sedan left the road at a high rate of speed, rolled over, and came to rest on its roof. What would be the best approach to gain access to the driver entrapped in the car?

A. Cut through the floor.

B. Open the doors or crawl through the windows.

C. Roll the car back over and then open the doors.

D. Use a wrecker wench to lift the car off its top.

44. When called to an accident scene involving a spill of hazardous materials, what should you do first?

A. Park the ambulance upwind from the accident scene, avoiding low areas.

B. Notify the local disaster management services prior to arrival.

C. Stop at a safe distance and scan the scene with binoculars.

D. Do a complete examination of any patients before moving them in case fractures are present.

45. Select the appropriate sequence for extricating a patient from an automobile.

    (1) Stabilize the vehicle.
    (2) Disentangle the patient.
    (3) Gain access.
    (4) Stabilize the patient.

    A. 1, 3, 4, 2.
    B. 1, 2, 3, 4.
    C. 3, 1, 4, 2.
    D. 3, 4, 1, 2.

46. You respond to a traffic accident on a freeway and detect a strong odor of gasoline. The local fire agency and state highway patrol arrive simultaneously. As a paramedic, what is your first responsibility on the scene?

    A. Patient care.
    B. Personal safety.
    C. Preservation of the scene.
    D. Gasoline washdown.

47. You and your EMT partner have been dispatched to a van versus pickup truck collision involving five persons. Passengers from the van are Patients #1 through #3. Patient #1 is the 36-year-old driver who was ejected on impact and is pulseless and apneic. Patient #2 is a 4-year-old child in a child restraint seat in the front passenger compartment. The child is crying, and the dash is embedded in her legs. Patient #3 is a 34-year-old female sitting behind the driver's seat. She is unresponsive and snoring. Patient #4 is the 21-year-old driver of the truck and is complaining of severe chest and upper abdominal pain. Patient #5, a passenger in the truck, is an 85-year-old female who presents with forehead abrasions, lip laceration, and disorientation. Initial triage of these patients is correctly identified as:

    A. Patients #1, #3, #4, #5, and #2.
    B. Patients #2, #1, #3, #4 and #5.
    C. Patients #3, #4, #5, #2, and #1.
    D. Patients #3, #4 #2, #1, and #5.

48. Your unit is the first to arrive after the crash of a commercial aircraft. You assume the role of command and size up the scene. There were 275

passengers and crew on departure. Communication with dispatch should be accomplished on:

A. The area's mutual frequency.
B. An assigned incident frequency.
C. The designed medical frequency.
D. A statewide UHF or VHF channel.

Stress Management

49. Which of the following is the *least* useful technique in the management of critical incident stress?

A. Demobilization.
B. Defusing.
C. Debriefing.
D. Incident critique.

50. A paramedic co-worker was the incident commander of a restaurant fire which resulted in 75 fatalities and 150 critically injured people. Although he has refused to discuss the incident in the following ten months, he has been aloof, irritable, jumpy, and complains of interrupted sleep. Both his and your units have been dispatched to a nursing home because the fire alarm has sounded. After arriving at the scene, he tells your crew to check the restaurant area for possible victims. You would recognize his behavior as that consistent with:

A. Critical incident stress.
B. Post-traumatic stress disorder.
C. Stress induced psychosis.
D. Cumulative stress disorder.

51. Your paramedic partner has been trying to earn extra money to buy a new car. He is working all of the overtime that is made available to him. Since the service is short-staffed at the present time, he frequently works 36 consecutive hours in the busiest district before taking 16 hours off. On your next duty shift, he complains of muscle aches, sore throat, and nausea. What is the basis for his complaints?

A. Direct patient contact on a continual basis increases pathogenic exposure, which constantly overwhelms the immune system.
B. Poor personal hygiene because he does not wash his hands or the ambulance equipment between patients.

C. Lack of sleep inhibits the functional ability of most cells involved with the immune system.

D. Stress increases cortisol serum secretion from the adrenal cortex, depressing the immune response.

52. On your last duty day, the son of a crew member was arrested for driving under the influence. During the next shift, your unit responds to an MVA involving an intoxicated youth. Before leaving the Emergency Department, the crew member begins to shout and lecture the injured youth's father. The crew member's behavior is consistent with which psychological defense mechanism?

A. Reaction formation.
B. Substitution.
C. Projection.
D. Sublimation.

53. Reactions to death and dying have been extensively researched over the past 20 years. What is the usual sequence of responses?

(1) Anger.
(2) Denial.
(3) Acceptance.
(4) Depression.
(5) Bargaining.

A. 1, 2, 4, 5, 3.
B. 2, 1, 5, 4, 3.
C. 3, 5, 2, 1, 4.
D. 4, 3, 5, 2, 1.

Answers with Rationale

1. (C) All of the information listed is important for effective emergency medical dispatch. However, crisis may cause confusion for the caller. Therefore, it is critical to obtain a telephone number that may be called in the event a caller hangs up the phone or gives erroneous information.

2. (C) The delegation of patient care responsibilities by the paramedic to the Basic EMT is acceptable and necessary in many situations. However, the paramedic may not authorize the EMT to perform any skills that are beyond the identified basic skill level.

3. (A) Ultimate responsibility for patient care rests with the base station physician, according to national standards. The paramedic, as the person present with the highest level of medical training, is responsible for implementation of the directions from the hospital base station. Local standards, however, may supersede the national standard, and you must be certain that you are clearly and currently informed on this issue.

4. (B) Certification verifies that an individual or agency has attained a predetermined level of competency. Licensure is the actual permission to practice. Credentialing is the verification of stated credentials.

5. (C) Professional competence, achieved by maintaining a high standard of training, is your best protection against the threat of being named as a defendant in a negligence case. Constant updating, with frequent continuing education, is a necessary part of a profession that is advancing rapidly. Malpractice insurance does not protect you from liability, although it can help provide for the fees incurred to prepare your defense, as well as funds for any judgment that might be awarded against you.

6. (B) You are legally responsible for any procedural errors, no matter how minor. You must report the dosage error. The health care practitioner must always double check the medication and prescribed dosage before administration. Additionally, when using a preloaded syringe, it is a good idea to evacuate any medication not intended for administration, prior to the injection. This practice reduces the chance of medication errors.

7. (D) Although KKK-A-1822 standardized ambulance design in 1974, improvement of ambulance electrical systems was accomplished in the 1980 revision (KKK-A-1822-A). In 1985, KKK-A-1822-B provided for implementation of standards from the National Institute for Occupational Safety and Health. The combined provisions are intended to improve ambulance function, reliability, and safety.

8. (A) It is imperative that paramedics and other EMS system personnel maintain the support of the entire medical community. This type of situation requires you to consider how your actions affect both in the present case and in the future. Allowing the physician to speak with Medical Control will provide an opportunity for you to continue patient care while the physician receives clarification on the local protocols.

9. (A) Off-line, or indirect, Medical Control allows the Medical Director to direct patient care through established protocols. On-line Medical Control involves radio or telephone communication for direct medical guidance. Quality assurance, a form of off-line Medical Control, is a process of retrospective case review to ensure that appropriate intervention was made and to promote continued improvement in the delivery of patient care.

10. (C) Although separate from issues of morality, professional ethics establish standards of rightness and wrongness for human conduct in a profession. It is not ethical for EMS personnel to express to a patient an opinion concerning a facility's real or perceived faults.

11. (B) Type III has a passageway between the driver's and patient's compartments while Type I does not. Although most have a raised roof, Type II ambulances are van-type design without access from the driver's compartment to the patient care area. Any ambulance certified as Type I, II, or III design may display the "Star of Life" symbol registered by the USDOT's National Highway Traffic Safety Administration (NHTSA).

12. (D) Good Samaritan laws are designed to afford legal protection for individuals at the scene of an emergency who assist in good faith, within their scope of practice, and without negligence. Although the primary intent of this legislation is universal, coverage (e.g., physician, nurse, EMS personnel) and circumstance (e.g., paid versus unpaid status) may

vary from state to state. These laws may be used for your defense, but most jurisdictions are moving away from the doctrine of immunity toward imposition of responsibility.

13. (C) Pregnancy and/or marriage entitle this patient to make decisions about her health care because she is legally an emancipated minor. As in any case involving refusal of treatment and/or transport, the consequences of refusal must be clearly communicated to the patient so that the decision is informed. A release form should be signed and must be witnessed. It is best to have someone else at the scene, other than a crew member, witness the signature to remove doubt of conspiracy should legal action be taken in the future. Should the patient refuse to sign, the refusal must be documented and witnessed in the same manner.

14. (A) Treatment without consent could be grounds for a battery lawsuit, but not for a negligence (error in treatment) suit. In order for a negligence case to be successfully tried, four components must be present: (1) duty: a relationship established between the paramedic and the patient; (2) breach of duty: the paramedic's failure to provide the type of care that a reasonably prudent person with similar training would provide; (3) proximate cause: what the paramedic did or did not do could *foreseeably* cause injury or damage to the patient; and (4) damages: actual damage or injury suffered by the patient as a result of the paramedic's failure to act as a prudent person with similar education and experience would have in the same situation.

15. (B) If you did not document application of a traction splint to the closed femur fracture, the court will consider that it was not done. At this point, the burden of proof rests on you, and a simple "I know I did it" will not be enough. Complete medical records must reflect care rendered as well as care not rendered, if that care might normally be expected. Due to the lapse of time, testimony from both your partner and you is highly questionable. What made this case so unique that your memories are so exact after all the runs you both have made since then? An audio cassette could have been made at any time and would not be credible evidence.

16. (A) The unconscious patient is treated by virtue of implied consent. The law assumes that if the patient knew he were in a life-threatening situation and could communicate, he would want you to intervene to counteract the threat to his life. Once the immediate life threat has passed, *or*

the patient regains consciousness, you must obtain voluntary consent. Expressed consent, the most preferred form, is conveyed by words or actions. Involuntary consent applies to situations where the patient is under the care of a guardian or guarantor, or cases involving an individual with Alzheimer's disease, one who has been declared mentally incompetent, or a patient under the custody of a law enforcement officer. Voluntary consent–special circumstances applies to a minor who does not need parental consent due to such circumstances as emancipated minor status, pregnancy, military service, or being a victim of child abuse.

17. (D) As an adult, this patient can withdraw consent that he has previously given. A patient's rights must be scrupulously upheld. You must make every effort possible, however, to convince him to allow you to treat. Once you have fully informed him of the possible consequences of his refusal, you must get him to sign a release form, unless injury precludes obtaining his signature. The next step is to objectively document his refusal of treatment, witnessed by a neutral party if possible.

18. (A) An act of omission is the failure to do that which a reasonably prudent person with the same or similar training would have done in the same or similar circumstances. An act of commission is engaging in a practice which a reasonably prudent person would not have done under the same or similar circumstances. Acts of omission (e.g., failure to secure the cervical spine) are more prevalent in lawsuits than those of commission.

19. (C) If you determine that Thelma is in control of her mental capacities, only the court can order that she be transported to the hospital Emergency Department. Medical Control (your Emergency Department physician), her son, and/or her physician cannot have her transported against her will, as there would be a chance of false imprisonment charges.

20. (B) One of the more common cases of abandonment occurs when a paramedic delivers the patient to the E.D. and leaves before giving report or before the E.D. nurse or physician has released the paramedic. In the event of a possible mass casualty situation, patient care responsibilities must be transferred as quickly as possible without compromising continued care. Although this may have been an interfacility transfer,

your responsibility to ensure uninterrupted patient care remains unchanged.

21. (D) Do not breach the patient's confidentiality. Your best response is to refer all media representatives to the spokesperson for the hospital.

22. (A) In order to treat a minor, you should obtain consent for treatment from one parent. If the child has a life-threatening condition and you are unable to contact a parent, implied consent applies. Should a conflict arise between parents, you may still treat the child; however, if you have time, it may be better to explain the medical consequences of delaying treatment to the recalcitrant party. Should both parents refuse consent, you cannot treat the child. Report your findings (facts and observations only) to the emergency department physician, police, or state child services division.

23. (C) All states have laws obligating health care providers, among others, to report cases of suspected child abuse or neglect to the appropriate authorities. The method of reporting involves completion of a written statement that is submitted to the investigative agency. Merely confiding your concerns or suspicions to the emergency department physician is insufficient action and does not relieve you of your legal responsibility. Subjective opinions should not be documented on the ambulance report form because such statements may be judged as libel if entered as evidence in a court.

24. (B) The unlawful touching of an individual without his consent poses a risk of being charged with battery. If a patient refuses a specific treatment, you should explain the potential consequences of such refusal. After you are assured his refusal is informed, you must notify Medical Control, document the incident on the report form, and proceed with transport. Negligence would not be incurred in this case of refusal unless the potential risks of refusing treatment were not explained to the patient. Care provided to a patient in a manner that violates a specified standard of care (e.g., CPR with a pulse present) is a type of negligence referred to as malfeasance. Assault exists when a situation results in a real or perceived threat of bodily harm to the patient.

25. (A) Correction of a legal document is usually accomplished by drawing a single line through the error followed by the initials of the person writ-

ing the report. Voiding the entire form is not an acceptable approach because such action creates doubt about when and why the form was changed. Liquid correction fluid and complete obliteration of the error are legally unacceptable because they lend an appearance of alteration.

26. (A) Unless a legal living will or valid DNR order exists, the paramedic must follow accepted standards of patient care. Chemical resuscitation in the absence of airway and dysrhythmia management amounts to negligence. Public education programs can help prevent calls to EMS in these situations.

27. (D) A duty to act requires the provider to respond to all calls within an identified response area. However, once a call has been accepted, there is also a duty to act. Failure to respond and deliver patient care would be judged as negligence and abandonment because the patient was not afforded ample opportunity to secure alternative health care.

28. (D) It is important for EMS personnel to recognize that a Do Not Resuscitate (DNR) order does not mean "Do Not Treat." This patient presents with a history and physical findings of severe dehydration. As a paramedic, you are required to administer the same standard of care to this patient as you would to a patient without a DNR order. Failure to do so could be construed as negligence. In the case of cardiac arrest, a DNR order can be troublesome for EMS providers. The local protocols should address the issue of DNR orders.

29. (C) Many states have enacted "living will" or "natural death request" legislation. If such legislation exists in your state, you should honor the request. It is imperative for EMS personnel to know what laws exist in respective areas of practice. Although the family's request for EMS is questionable, you should support them during this crisis and contact the appropriate authorities for them. However, if in doubt about the document or persons making the decision, follow the AHA recommendations and err on the side of resuscitation.

30. (A) It is important to transmit data in a priority order, because it allows the physician to more rapidly diagnose the problem and plan the appropriate treatment. Age and sex are communicated first in order to identify the patient category (pediatric, adult, or geriatric). Vital signs follow because they vary with age and immediately reflect possible pathology (hypertension, hypotension, tachycardia, bradycardia, hyperpnea,

hypopnea, tachypnea, bradypnea, etc.). The chief complaint is given third because it is the reason the patient or bystander summoned help and often adds definition to the vital signs. Additional pertinent information should be communicated in a concise, organized sequence (history of present illness, physical findings, past medical history, allergies, medications, etc.).

31. (D) No funding is provided by the Federal Communications Commission (FCC), which was established as a regulatory and controlling agency. Frequency and license regulations originated with the FCC, and enforcement of the regulations is its responsibility. Therefore, the FCC conducts spot checks of base stations and monitors frequencies in order to fulfill this responsibility.

32. (C) A duplex communication system uses two frequencies. The field can transmit voice or telemetry on one frequency and simultaneously receive hospital orders on another frequency. A half-duplex communication system employs one radio frequency that allows field transmission of either voice or telemetry to the hospital base station at any given time. The field cannot receive a transmission while transmitting voice or telemetry. A simplex system is composed of a single one-way frequency.

33. (D) Sixty-cycle alternating current produces these characteristic waves and spikes in the ECG transmission due to the intermittent surge of power associated with alternating current. The weakening of transmitter power causes dwarfing of the ECG waveforms which prevents the distinction among the markings. Patient muscle tremors cause sharp spiking that does not have a uniform configuration like that of sixty-cycle interference. Loose patient ECG electrodes cause a wandering baseline, giving the tracing a "roller coaster" appearance.

34. (A) The repeater retransmits the mobile unit's signal on another frequency, thus increasing the signal range. An encoder is used with a decoder to prevent unnecessary reception of transmissions intended for another base station. Resembling a telephone dial, the encoder transmits a pulsed tone that is received at the base station by the decoder. Although several base stations may operate on the same radio frequency, the decoder responds only to an assigned three- or four-digit pulsed tone. An acoustic coupler allows the transmission of telemetry over the radio by joining the radio to the telephone hand piece.

35. (D) A remote console is a control console that is connected to the base station by telephone lines. An encoder resembles a telephone dial that causes pulsed tones to be sent out over the air when dialed. A repeater receives a signal on one frequency and retransmits that signal on another frequency. A decoder-equipped receiver responds only to an individually programmed code.

36. (C) All of the components listed are necessary components for an effective Emergency Medical Services communication network. Entrance into the system requires rapid citizen access as well as efficient dispatch. Medical Control is delivered via hospital-to-field and field-to-hospital communications. Interhospital communications are especially necessary in situations involving mass casualties.

37. (C) Transmission of a signal over water increases the range of a mobile transmitter/receiver.

38. (A) Satellite receivers ensure that a lower-power unit will always be within range of the system. Satellite receivers are connected to the repeater by dedicated telephone lines or microwave relay. An encoder resembles a telephone dial or the buttons of a push-button telephone. When activated, the encoder sends pulses or tones over the air. Receivers with decoders can recognize these codes or tones. When a decoder receives the correct code, the audio circuits of the receiver are activated. Remote consoles extend all operating controls to a remote site and are connected to the base station by dedicated telephone lines, microwave, or other radios.

39. (D) The dispatcher must gather essential information prior to dispatching the vehicle. Although the vehicle may be dispatched as soon as the location and nature of the call are received, the dispatcher must obtain the caller's name, a call-back number, and address of the event. The patient's past medical history has no relevance to the dispatch of the vehicle. ALS versus BLS decisions are made on the basis of the nature of the call.

40. (C) Speaking at close range improves the clarity of transmission to the base station. While the paramedic should keep the voice free from emotion, a normal pitch—not monotone—should be used. In order to prevent simultaneous transmissions on a single frequency, the paramedic

should listen to a channel before transmitting to make certain that it is not in use by another unit at that time.

41. (D) The telephone provides the highest level of privacy for communications since telephone messages are not transmitted over the airways. The patient's name should not be stated until arrival at the hospital in any type of communication. The "echo" procedure is used to prevent any type of misunderstanding regarding orders (i.e., repeating an order prior to completing it).

42. (B) The Kendricks Extrication Device (KED) is the most appropriate device from the listed alternatives for spinal immobilization prior to moving the patient onto a long backboard. A Cervical Immobilization Device (CID) is attached to a long backboard for additional cervical immobilization. The scoop stretcher is designed to slide under a patient lying supine on a surface without moving the patient first.

43. (B) Access to a patient trapped in an overturned car may be gained by crawling through windows or opening doors. The floor would be extremely difficult to cut through. Keep in mind that access is only necessary to allow you to examine and treat a patient. A large opening can later be developed for the extrication phase. Never roll a car back over.

44. (C) Prior to involving your vehicle, crew, and person in a hazardous material scene, you need to identify potential dangers as well as the substance, if possible. Vehicles transporting such chemicals are required to display placards for product identification. Whereas most haulers comply with federal law, some do not, thus compounding your problems. Use of binoculars is the *first* step in managing a hazardous material situation because substance identification is often possible from a safe distance. This prevents unnecessary exposure and additional risk. Although the scene should be approached upwind, avoiding low-lying areas, this is *not* the first action to be taken. Patent care occurs only *after* rescuer safety is ensured.

45. (A) No patient contact is made until the scene and vehicle are secured. After safety priorities are addressed, rescuers can gain access in order to begin patient care. Once the patient is stabilized (e.g., cervical spine, airway, etc.), disentanglement is accomplished. Depending on the com-

plexity of the situation, this may be a lengthy process requiring EMS personnel to deliver more extensive patient care (e.g., IV fluids, medications, etc.).

46. (B) Your first responsibility is to assure personal safety, so that you will be available to provide patient care. The strong odor of gasoline causes you to be concerned about the possibility of an explosion. You should proceed with patient care once the scene is declared safe. The other trained professionals on the scene are responsible for preservation of the scene and gasoline washdown, if necessary.

47. (C) Triage, or sorting, is a continuous process based on assessment and patient status. Initial triage decisions must be made on the basis of severity and survivability with given resources. Patient #3 must have immediate airway management if she is to survive. Patient #4 has potential chest injuries decreasing ventilatory status, and abdominal injuries that can result in extensive internal hemorrhage. Patient #5 has a head injury that presents potential airway complications. Patient #2 has a patent airway and is breathing, as indicated by crying. Patient #1 cannot be resuscitated at this time due to lack of appropriate resources. If resuscitation is initiated, there is no one to manage the living patients. Once additional resources arrive, resuscitation can be undertaken.

48. (B) Assuming the role of incident commander in a major incident response requires you to provide control and direction necessary to coordinate resources into and out of the scene. Using a preassigned incident frequency lets all responders know that command has been established. This action also helps prevent confusion and communication system overload. It is important for an area disaster plan to include this frequency designation for all services within the plan and all those that offer mutual aid.

49. (D) An incident critique is a cognitive (intellectual) review of the event. It generally does not encourage or allow for expression of the emotions, reactions, and signs and symptoms of the acute stress response. Demobilizations, defusings, and debriefings have all proven to reduce the harmful effects of stress and accelerate recovery in normal people having normal reactions to abnormal events.

50. (B) Post-traumatic stress disorder (PTSD) has many physical, emotional, and psychological manifestations which may persist for more

than one month. This paramedic's signs and symptoms, as well as duration, are consistent with PTSD. In addition, the nursing home incident caused him to experience a flashback due to situational similarities. This condition is not psychotic behavior, but the mind's attempt
to work through a terrible experience which has been suppressed due
to an enormous amount of pain associated with it. The paramedic in
this situation urgently needs evaluation and possible assistance in
overcoming the stress and possible sense of guilt due to a perceived
failure.

51. (D) When the body is exposed to stress, it attempts to protect itself
against injury. Part of this response is to prevent inflammatory reactions
(e.g., ulceration of the gastric mucosa due to increased acidity). The adrenal cortex secretes corticosteroids that cause anti-inflammatory responses. Since the immune system is involved in the events resulting in
inflammation, its activities are also suppressed. Thus, the stressed individual, while being protected against the adverse effects of stress, is also
highly susceptible to infection from microorganisms.

52. (C) Defense mechanisms are normal adaptive functions of personality that assist in adjusting to stressful situations. They become patho-
logical only if used excessively to avoid reality. Projection is attribut-
ing to another person or object those thoughts, feelings, motives, or
desires that are really one's own unacceptable traits. Reaction formation involves overt behavior or attitudes that are the exact opposite of
underlying unacceptable impulses. Substitution is the replacement of
an unattainable or unacceptable activity by one that is attainable or
acceptable. It may also be expressed by redirecting an emotion from
the original object to a more acceptable substitute object. Sublimation
is the diversion of unacceptable, instinctual drives into socially acceptable channels.

53. (B) The initial response is denial, a temporary defense common to almost everyone. Then the patient or family may express anger over the
loss. Bargaining is an attempt to enter into some type of agreement with
God, or another superior being, in hopes of postponing the inevitable.
The last stage, acceptance, occurs when the person and/or family ac-
cepts the inevitable. However, these stages may vary from person to
person and are subject to change. In other words, a patient may demonstrate acceptance one day and bargaining the next. This is a dynamic
process.

3

Preparatory

General Patient Assessment

1. When measuring the diastolic blood pressure, you are evaluating the:

   A. Total peripheral resistance to blood flow.
   B. Amount of pressure during left ventricular contraction.
   C. Difference between ventricular contraction and relaxation.
   D. Pulse pressure as reflected through resting cardiac output.

2. An 81-year-old male fell down two steps. You examine him and determine he has a fractured hip. Your conclusion is based on the shortening and abduction of the leg. The abducted position of the leg indicates a position:

   A. Opposite of the anatomical position.
   B. Proximal to the midsagittal plane.
   C. Away from the body's midline.
   D. With exaggerated rigidity and extension.

3. A 4-year-old boy fell off a porch approximately five minutes prior to your arrival. During the physical examination, you note the child has a humeral deformity. When you bring the patient into the emergency room, the physician tells you he suspects the patient sustained a fracture in the growth section of the bone. You would recognize that section as the:

   A. Ginglymus.
   B. Diaphysis.
   C. Epiphysis.
   D. Periosteum.

4. When describing a patient's respiratory status and level of consciousness, the paramedic is most correct by giving the following report:

   A. The patient appears somewhat confused at this time and is unable to communicate effectively. His respirations appear labored.
   B. The patient has periods of rapid, irregular breaths alternating with periods of apnea and has no response to verbal or painful stimuli.
   C. The patient is breathing fast and then slow at about 10 respirations per minute and appears lethargic. He is unable to communicate.
   D. The patient is experiencing periods of apnea that alternate with periods of rapid, irregular breathing and is in a semi-comatose state.

5. The *least* valuable information to obtain when taking a patient history is:

   A. Allergies.
   B. Family history.
   C. Current medications.
   D. Underlying medical problems.

6. Evaluation of which of the following is *not* part of the primary survey?

   A. Circulation.
   B. Hemorrhage.
   C. Vital signs.
   D. Level of consciousness.

7. In general, the "chief complaint" may be characterized as:

   A. The patient's presenting symptom.
   B. The paramedic's diagnosis.
   C. The objective data revealed by the physical exam.
   D. The physician's evaluation of the patient's problem.

8. Which of the following conditions cause dilation of the pupils?

   (1) Fright.
   (2) Pain.
   (3) Parasympathetic stimulation.
   (4) Hypoxemia.

   A. 1, 2, 4.
   B. 2, 3, 4.
   C. 1, 2, 3.
   D. 1, 3, 4.

9. During your examination of an 87-year-old male involved in a vehicular accident, you note that when his right eye looks forward, his left eye looks outward. This sign is known as:

   A. Racoon's eyes.
   B. Doll's eyes.
   C. Dysconjugate gaze.
   D. Battle's sign.

10. During a baseball game, a foul ball strikes a 17-year-old spectator in her right occipital region. She is alert and can communicate. She is complaining of partial loss of vision in both eyes and pain at the point of impact. Upon examination, the paramedic finds an ecchymotic area at the point of impact, but no open wound. No other signs of injury are noted, and the vital signs are within normal limits. Why does the patient suffer from partial loss of vision in both eyes?

    A. The vision loss must be due to another undiscovered injury, as the right side of the brain controls the left side of the body.
    B. The vision loss occurs because some of the injured optic nerve fibers cross from the right to the left side of the body.
    C. The vision loss is due to a contrecoup injury to the left eye.
    D. None of the above can explain the observed partial loss of vision.

11. Tapping of body surfaces to elicit changes in sound is called:

    A. Inspection.
    B. Auscultation.
    C. Palpation.
    D. Percussion.

12. An 18-year-old female patient complains of abdominal pain, but denies nausea, vomiting, or diarrhea. She also denies the possibility of pregnancy. These denials are known as:

    A. Abnormal signs.
    B. Pertinent negatives.
    C. Normal symptoms.
    D. Chief complaints.

13. Which of the following devices is capable of delivering the highest oxygen concentration?

    A. Simple face mask.
    B. Nonrebreathing mask.
    C. Nasal cannula.
    D. Venturi mask.

14. What is the most serious drawback of using positive pressure/demand valves?

A. Lung compliance cannot be felt.
B. High airway pressures are created.
C. They consume a tremendous supply of oxygen.
D. They depend on a power source.

15. When you are ventilating an nonbreathing adult patient, the minimum ventilation volume required is:

A. 500 cc.
B. 800 cc.
C. 1000 cc.
D. 1200 cc.

16. When you are inserting an esophageal obturator airway device, the patient's head should be in which position?

A. Hyperextended.
B. Sniff position.
C. Neutral or flexed position.
D. Hyperextended or neutral position.

17. Which statement about the esophageal obturator airway (EOA) is most correct?

A. The EOA lessens the likelihood of regurgitation of stomach contents.
B. EOA ventilation is superior to bag-valve-mask ventilation.
C. The EOA provides an open airway.
D. The EOA provides a better mask seal than other devices.

18. All of the following statements about the pocket mask are true *except*:

A. It is the preferred method of BLS ventilation.
B. At flow rates of 10 L/min, 50% oxygen may be delivered.
C. It may be used as a simple oxygen face mask.
D. It delivers smaller tidal volumes than a BVM.

19. While eating, a restaurant patron suddenly cannot speak, stops breathing, and grabs at his throat. Your initial efforts at abdominal thrusts are unsuccessful, and the patient remains conscious. You should:

A. Attempt transtracheal jet insufflation.
B. Continue the abdominal thrusts.

C. Attempt finger sweeps.

D. Attempt to push the object down his right bronchus.

20. Skin color changes in a dark-skinned person can be observed in the:

A. Mouth.
B. Axilla.
C. Ears.
D. Feet.

21. James Logan is a 53-year-old male who has fallen from a ladder and sustained a deep laceration to his thigh. Bright red blood is spurting from the wound. In preparing to treat James, you recall the correct sequence for controlling bleeding, which is:

A. Direct pressure, pressure points, tourniquets.
B. Pressure points, direct pressure, tourniquets.
C. Tourniquets, direct pressure, pressure points.
D. Pressure points, tourniquets, direct pressure.

22. When evaluating an extremity for injury, you may need to use terms describing range of motion. The term *abduction* means that the extremity is moved:

A. Forward.
B. Backward.
C. Toward the body.
D. Away from the body.

23. The hamstring muscle is an example of which type of muscle group?

A. Flexor.
B. Extensor.
C. Pronator.
D. Supinator.

24. Approximately how far should a nasogastric tube be advanced in the average patient?

A. 10 inches.
B. 15 inches.
C. 20 inches.
D. 35 inches.

25. Select the equipment needed for performing nasogastric tube insertion in a conscious patient.

    A. Levine tube, 50-cc syringe, and cup of water with straw.
    B. Vasoline lubricant, Levine tube, and cup of water with straw.
    C. 50-cc syringe, Levine tube, and Vasoline lubricant.
    D. Cup of water with straw, Levine tube, Vasoline lubricant, and 50-cc syringe.

Airway and Ventilation

26. The EOA is contraindicated in all cases *except* those involving:

    A. A foreign body in the airway.
    B. An elderly patient over age 65.
    C. A patient under age 16.
    D. A patient under 5 feet tall.

27. The straight laryngoscope blade is inserted:

    A. Anterior to the epiglottis.
    B. Posterior to the epiglottis.
    C. Into the esophagus.
    D. Between the vocal cords.

28. The first bifurcation of the trachea produces:

    A. Two bronchi, of which the left is longer and has a more acute angle than the right.
    B. Two bronchi, of which the right is longer and has a more acute angle than the left.
    C. Three bronchi, of which the medial is longer and has a less acute curve than the left or right.
    D. Two bronchi, equal in length and angulation.

29. Which of the following statements about suction procedure is *incorrect*?

    A. The primary complication of endotracheal suctioning is hypoxia.
    B. A 15-second limitation for tracheal suction reduces potential complications.
    C. The suction unit should provide a vacuum in excess of 30 mm Hg when the tube is clamped.
    D. After inserting the catheter into the endotracheal tube, suction is applied while rotating the catheter as it is removed.

30. An adequate bag-valve-mask unit should include all of the following criteria *except*:

    A. Oxygen inlet and reservoir system.
    B. A true nonrebreathing valve.
    C. Pop-off valves on pediatric sizes.
    D. A nonjam valve system at 15 liters oxygen per minute.

31. What is the required patient position necessary for optimal visualization of the vocal cords during endotracheal intubation?

    A. Chin to chest.
    B. Neck hyperextended and forehead tilted back.
    C. Head turned to the left and tilted forward.
    D. Neck flexed forward and head extended backward.

32. When auscultating for correct EOA or ET placement, the paramedic should listen over the:

    A. Larynx and both lungs.
    B. Epigastrium and both lungs.
    C. Right and left lungs.
    D. Epigastrium and left lung.

33. The inferior portion of the larynx is formed by the:

    A. Cricoid cartilage.
    B. Arytenoid cartilage.
    C. Thyroid cartilage.
    D. Hyoid bone.

34. You have rescued a 10-year-old child from a backyard swimming pool. None of the bystanders know how long the child was submerged. After establishing a patent airway, you note that the child is breathing and has a pulse. During the secondary assessment, you find the chest is clear with equal breath sounds. What is the physiological basis for this clinical finding?

    A. Protective mechanism provided by the gag reflex.
    B. Sustained spasm involving the true vocal cords.

C. Water aspiration confined to the bronchi.

D. Contraction of the false vocal cords.

35. Endotracheal intubation using the MacIntosh blade requires you to position the tip of the blade into the:

A. Nasopharynx.

B. Vallecula.

C. Oropharynx.

D. Epiglottis.

36. After correctly positioning the endotracheal tube, you inflate the cuff. The primary reason for inflating the cuff is to:

A. Stabilize the position of the tube.

B. Prevent aspiration of foreign material.

C. Allow direct ventilation with 100% oxygen.

D. Decrease the incidence of gastric distention.

37. After inserting the pharyngeal-tracheal lumen airway (PTLA), the paramedic provides ventilation into the short tube. If there is no chest wall movement or audible breath sound, the paramedic should:

A. Remove the stylet from the long tube.

B. Suction the short tube and then attempt to ventilate.

C. Inflate the distal cuff until ventilations are apparent.

D. Withdraw the airway and hyperventilate the patient with oxygen.

38. Other than the number of tubes and inflatable cuffs, the significant difference between the pharyngeal-tracheal lumen airway (PTLA) and the esophageal obturator airway (EOA) is that the PTLA does *not*:

A. Occlude the esophagus when inserted correctly.

B. Require direct visualization.

C. Indirectly ventilate the lungs.

D. Require the use of a face mask.

39. Your patient is a 23-year-old male with a gunshot wound to the right lateral chest. Assessment reveals a patent airway, inadequate respiratory efforts, and a rapid thready pulse. After inserting the laryngoscope,

your paramedic partner directs your attention to the monitor which demonstrates the following ECG:

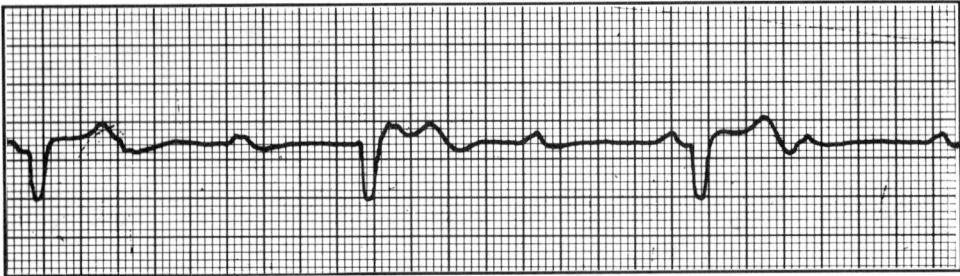

You would:

A. Inform your partner that this is a normal consequence of endotracheal intubation.
B. Remove the laryngoscope and hyperventilate the patient with 100% oxygen before any further attempts.
C. Direct your partner to administer atropine sulfate 0.5 mg IV and repeat the dose in 5 minutes if needed.
D. Discontinue the intubation procedure and insert the esophageal obturator airway for rapid airway procurement.

40. The primary reason for performing the Sellick maneuver is to:

A. Align the vocal cords and make intubation easier.
B. Prevent regurgitation during ventilation or intubation.
C. Prevent hyperextension of the head during intubation.
D. Align the pharynx to make EOA placement easier.

41. The technique of blind nasotracheal intubation is absolutely or potentially contraindicated in which of the following situations?

(1) Apneic trauma patient in need of intubation.
(2) Breathing patient with massive maxillofacial trauma.
(3) Responsive patient in respiratory failure.
(4) Breathing trauma patient with possible cervical spine injury.

A. 1, 4.
B. 2, 3.
C. 1, 2.
D. 1, 3.

42. You are treating a 45-year-old, unresponsive, apneic, trauma patient who has hemorrhage into the airway with resulting airway compromise. The preferred method of airway control is:

    A. Pharyngeal-tracheal lumen airway.
    B. Nasotracheal intubation with neutral alignment of the spine.
    C. Orotracheal intubation with neutral alignment of the spine.
    D. Esophageal obturator airway.

43. When intubating a child, you should use an uncuffed endotracheal tube for which of the following reasons?

    A. The pressure of a standard ET tube cuff would injure the trachea.
    B. A child is less likely to regurgitate and aspirate stomach contents.
    C. An uncuffed tube fits snugly through the glottic opening.
    D. An uncuffed tube fits snugly through the cricoid cartilage.

44. When you are performing percutaneous transtracheal jet insufflation, which of the following are necessary for adequate ventilation?

    (1) Catheter of at least 14 gauge.
    (2) 30–50 psi manual jet ventilator.
    (3) Bag-valve-mask with reservoir and adapter.
    (4) Catheter of at least 20 gauge.

    A. 1, 2.
    B. 3, 4.
    C. 2, 4.
    D. 2, 3.

Pathophysiology of Shock

45. What is the most accurate definition of the shock state?

    A. The level of carbon dioxide in the blood exceeds 50 mm Hg.
    B. Oxygen and nutrients are not transported to the cells for use.
    C. Metabolic needs increase, and there is a concurrent decrease in body temperature.
    D. Cells lose permeability, and oxygen and nutrients cannot be transported into the cells.

46. You are called to the scene of a one-car MVA and find the two occupants have been thrown from their rolled vehicle. You examine an unconscious male who appears pale, cool to the touch, and sweaty. He has no major visible injuries. His pulse is 130 and BP is 92/60. You should treat this patient as though he were in:

    A. Hypovolemic shock.
    B. Neurogenic shock.
    C. Cardiogenic shock.
    D. Respiratory shock.

47. Decreased blood flow through the capillaries produces all of the following effects *except*:

    A. Conversion of cellular metabolism from aerobic to anaerobic.
    B. Change in capillary permeability.
    C. Increased red cell aggregation.
    D. Arterial pressure increases above 80 mm Hg.

48. Septic shock results from:

    A. Spinal cord injury.
    B. Internal hemorrhage.
    C. Infectious states.
    D. Cardiac disease states.

49. Cardiogenic shock occurs when the heart:

    A. Is not effective as a pump to meet the body's need for oxygen.
    B. Becomes ineffective due to a decreased circulatory blood volume.
    C. Does not adequately respond to stimulation by the sympathetic nervous system.
    D. Develops an obstruction, such as a large embolus.

50. When cellular oxygen perfusion is decreased:

    A. Capillaries rupture.
    B. ATP release is increased.
    C. Anaerobic metabolism occurs.
    D. Cells dehydrate.

51. The cool and pale skin of patients in shock results from:

    A. Generalized vasoconstriction.
    B. Loss of thermoregulatory mechanisms.

C. A vasovagal response to trauma.
D. Blood being shunted to the chest.

52. Hypovolemia occurs in conditions other than hemorrhage. An example is:

A. Pericardial tamponade.
B. Compartment syndrome.
C. Third space fluid loss.
D. Spinal cord injury.

53. When a patient exhibits distended jugular neck veins with vital sign changes representative of a shock state (increased pulse rate and decreased blood pressure), the distention is most likely caused by:

A. A ruptured sternocleidomastoid muscle.
B. Hypotension.
C. Dissecting thoracic aneurysm.
D. Tension pneumothorax.

54. A priority action in treating a patient for shock is to start an IV. The usual intravenous fluid replacement in hypovolemia is:

A. A dextrose solution.
B. A crystalloid solution.
C. A colloid solution.
D. Salt-poor albumin (25%).

55. Generalized shock occuring as a severe reaction to the ingestion or injection of an antigen is:

A. A vasovagal response.
B. A Voges-Proskauer reaction.
C. A normal response.
D. Anaphylactic shock.

56. Urine output decreases to less than 30 ml/hour in shock states as a result of:

A. Decreased blood flow through the kidneys.
B. Decreased blood flow through the abdominal organs.
C. The bladder's inability to contract.
D. Dehydration of the cells.

57. The cation that is primarily responsible for the regulation and distribution of water throughout the body is:

    A. Potassium.
    B. Calcium.
    C. Magnesium.
    D. Sodium.

58. Which statement is most correct about isotonic IV crystalloid solutions when 1000 cc are infused?

    A. 1000 cc stay in the vascular space.
    B. It carries oxygen and is a substitute for blood volume.
    C. 250 cc stay in the vascular space, and 750 cc leak to the interstitial space.
    D. 750 cc stay in the vascular space, and 250 cc leak to the interstitial space.

59. Which of the following solutions causes cells to expand by osmosis?

    A. Isotonic.
    B. Hypotonic.
    C. Hypertonic.
    D. Hydrostatic.

60. The primary difference between crystalloid and colloid solutions is that colloid solutions:

    A. Contain proteins and stay in the vascular space.
    B. Contain proteins and rapidly leave the vascular space.
    C. Contain large sugar molecules and act as an osmotic diuretic.
    D. Contain electrolytes and rapidly leave the vascular space.

61. An isotonic IV solution is one that has a solute concentration:

    A. Greater than that within the cell.
    B. Equal to that within the cell.
    C. Less than that within the cell.
    D. Twice the osmolarity of body cells.

62. Blood volume is equal to what percent of body weight?

    A. 3–4%.
    B. 4–6%.

C. 6–8%.
D. 8–10%.

63. Which of the following is the normal body pH?

A. 7.3 (7.25 to 7.35).
B. 7.4 (7.35 to 7.45).
C. 7.5 (7.45 to 7.55).
D. 7.6 (7.55 to 7.65).

64. The body's three mechanisms for the regulation of acid-base balance, from fastest to slowest, are:

A. Respiratory, buffer, kidneys.
B. Buffer, respiratory, kidneys.
C. Kidneys, buffer, respiratory.
D. Buffer, kidneys, respiratory.

65. When the buffer system absorbs hydrogen ions, the by-product is:

A. Calcium chloride.
B. Sodium chloride.
C. Carbonic acid.
D. Ascorbic acid.

66. In compensated hypovolemic shock, the first organ from which blood is diverted is the:

A. Brain.
B. Kidneys.
C. Liver.
D. Skin.

67. To compensate for blood or fluid loss, the baroreceptor response attempts to maintain blood pressure by:

A. Increased heart rate and vasodilation.
B. Decreased heart rate and vasoconstriction.
C. Increased heart rate and vasoconstriction.
D. Decreased heart rate and vasodilation.

68. Which of the following vital signs is *least* significant in early recognition of hypovolemic shock?

A. Blood pressure.
B. Pulse rate.
C. Capillary refill time.
D. Respiratory rate.

69. What percent of blood loss in a healthy patient is usually necessary to cause uncompensated shock?

   A. 10%.
   B. 20%.
   C. 30%.
   D. 40%.

70. Neurogenic shock is most often the result of:

   A. Head injury.
   B. Spinal cord injury.
   C. Syncope.
   D. Allergic reactions.

71. Patients in neurogenic shock usually have all of the following *except*:

   A. Hypotension.
   B. Tachycardia/vasoconstriction.
   C. Thirst.
   D. Increased respiratory rate.

72. You are treating a 20-year-old, unresponsive trauma patient whose head was struck when he fell from a ladder. He has no previous medical history and is not on any medication. His only obvious injury is a scalp laceration. His vital signs are P 50, R 20, BP 210/100. Based on this information, you should suspect:

   A. Neurogenic shock.
   B. Hypovolemic shock.
   C. Cardiogenic shock.
   D. Increased intracranial pressure.

73. What is one of the earliest complications of shock hypoperfusion?

   A. Adult respiratory distress syndrome.
   B. Acute renal failure.
   C. Acute hepatic failure.
   D. Transient ischemic attack.

A. Chronic obstructive pulmonary disease.
B. Gastroenteritis.
C. Chronic liver disease.
D. Cholecystitis.

83. Select the correct statement regarding subcutaneous injections:

    A. A subcutaneous injection is absorbed more rapidly than oral medication.
    B. One to five milliliters of solution may be administered by subcutaneous route.
    C. The needle is inserted at a 15- to 20-degree angle to the skin.
    D. The skin is stretched and held taut during a subcutaneous injection.

84. When the combined effect of drugs is greater than the sum of their individual effects, the action is known as:

    A. Cumulative action.
    B. Synergism.
    C. Hypersensitivity.
    D. Idiosyncrasy.

85. You are ordered to administer 1/8 grain morphine sulfate to a patient. The prefilled syringe contains 10 mg in 1 ml. How much morphine will you need to administer?

    A. 0.33 ml.
    B. 0.50 ml.
    C. 0.67 ml.
    D. 0.75 ml.

86. At the scene of a vehicular accident, you find an 18-year-old male who has signs and symptoms of internal injuries. Medical Control orders you to start an IV with a large-bore needle and administer fluid at the rate of 200 cc/hour. With an administration set of 15 gtts/cc, how many gtts per minute will the patient receive?

    A. 15 gtts/min.
    B. 30 gtts/min.
    C. 50 gtts/min.
    D. 60 gtts/min.

87. What are the two systems of measurement used to measure and dispense drugs?

    A. Apothecary and English.
    B. English and metric.
    C. Household and English.
    D. Apothecary and metric.

88. What is the rationale for pinching off intravenous tubing when administering IV medications?

    A. It prevents infusing the medication into the vein too rapidly.
    B. It prevents the medication from flowing up the tubing and becoming diluted with the solution.
    C. It causes the medication to flow into the vein and not up the IV tubing.
    D. It causes a positive osmotic gradient that increases the absorption of the medication.

89. What is the primary objective for stretching the skin while administering an intramuscular injection?

    A. Reducing the thickness of the subcutaneous tissues.
    B. Increasing the absorption of the medication.
    C. Permitting the needle to penetrate the skin more easily.
    D. Eliminating the possibility of injecting the medication directly into a blood vessel.

90. Emergency care is required for a 65-year-old male farmer who was poisoned while spraying insecticides. Which of the following is the *least* probable route of his exposure to the poison?

    A. Absorption.
    B. Injection.
    C. Inhalation.
    D. Ingestion.

91. Your patient is to receive a 4 mg/min infusion of lidocaine. What drip rate should you establish for a mixture of 1 gm of lidocaine in 0.25 L of 5% DW when using a microdrop administration set?

    A. 15 gtts/min.
    B. 30 gtts/min.

C. 45 gtts/min.
D. 60 gtts/min.

92. Which of the following routes is the least appropriate for medication administration in a prehospital setting?

    A. Oral.
    B. Sublingual.
    C. Subcutaneous.
    D. Intravenous.

93. Which of the following pharmaceutical preparations are generally indicated for external use?

    (1) Elixirs
    (2) Suppositories
    (3) Tinctures
    (4) Spirits
    (5) Lotions
    (6) Astringents

    A. 1, 3, 5, 6.
    B. 1, 2, 4.
    C. 2, 3, 4.
    D. 3, 5, 6.

94. When giving a drug in suspension form, the paramedic must always remember to:

    A. Have the patient's nose as close to the container as possible for maximal inhalation.
    B. Shake the container thoroughly so that the alcohol content is well distributed.
    C. Ensure the ingredients are well mixed by shaking the container.
    D. Tap the top of the container prior to opening it.

95. Intramuscular and subcutaneous injections are generally contraindicated for the patient who is:

    A. Experiencing respiratory distress.
    B. Cold, clammy, and pale.
    C. Complaining of pain.
    D. Obese.

96. The progressive diminution of susceptibility to the effects of a drug resulting from the drug's continued administration defines the term:

    A. Tolerance.
    B. Habituation.
    C. Untoward effect.
    D. Cumulative action.

97. While you are developing the history from your 37-year-old female patient, she tells you that she is allergic to sulfa drugs. When asked what she experiences when she takes sulfa compounds, she tells you that they make her extremely nauseous. This would indicate drug:

    A. Hypersensitivity.
    B. Potentiation.
    C. Side effect.
    D. Synergism.

98. If Medical Control orders a medication that is contraindicated for a patient, the paramedic should first:

    A. Refuse to administer the drug.
    B. Give the drug because the physician is liable for the order.
    C. Look up the drug in a reference for a double check.
    D. Question the order by repeating it before any other activity.

99. You have an order for 750 mg of a particular drug. If each tablet contains 0.5 gm, how many tablets would you administer?

    A. 1.5.
    B. 2.0.
    C. 2.5.
    D. 3.0.

100. You are ordered to add 150 mg of aminophylline to D_5W for a total volume of 100 ml. Aminophylline is available in a concentration of 0.5 gm in 0.02 liter. How many milliliters of aminophylline should you add to the IV solution?

    A. 6 ml.
    B. 8 ml.
    C. 12 ml.
    D. 16 ml.

101. You are ordered to infuse aminophylline over 20 minutes. If the drop factor is 10, you should regulate the IV infusion to how many gtts/min?

    A. 50 gtts/min.
    B. 55 gtts/min.
    C. 60 gtts/min.
    D. 65 gtts/min.

102. You are instructed to administer 30 mg of a drug that is in a concentration of 15 mg/0.5 ml. How many milliliters would be required to deliver the ordered dosage?

    A. 0.50 ml.
    B. 1.00 ml.
    C. 2.00 ml.
    D. 3.00 ml.

103. You are ordered to administer 0.01 mg/kg of a drug to a patient who weighs 165 pounds. If the medication is available in a 1:1000 solution, you should administer:

    A. 0.25 ml.
    B. 0.50 ml.
    C. 0.75 ml.
    D. 1.00 ml.

104. The paramedic must always observe safety precautions when administering medications to a patient. Which of the following is *not* consistent with safety precautions?

    A. Concentrating on the task itself.
    B. Following orders immediately after receiving them.
    C. Making sure that the physician's orders are understood.
    D. Relaying the list of current medications to Medical Control.

105. The appropriate needle gauge for administering a drug subcutaneously is:

    A. 25 gauge.
    B. 23 gauge.
    C. 21 gauge.
    D. 19 gauge.

106. The IM route of medication administration is often selected over the subcutaneous route for all of the following reasons *except*:

A. Rapidity of absorption.
B. Volume of medication that can be administered.
C. Nature of the medication to be administered.
D. Decreased possibility of other tissue damage.

107. Which of the following drugs are absorbed by the bronchial tree and can be administered via an endotracheal tube?

   (1) Verapamil.
   (2) Naloxone.
   (3) Atropine.
   (4) Diphenhydramine.
   (5) Lidocaine.
   (6) Epinephrine.

A. 1, 2 ,3 ,4.
B. 2, 3, 5, 6.
C. 1, 2, 5, 6.
D. 3, 4, 5, 6.

108. What is the recommended minimal volume of drugs administered via endotracheal tube?

A. 5 cc.
B. 10 cc.
C. 15 cc.
D. 20 cc.

109. A drug is described as having Beta-2 selective effects on the autonomic nervous system. In theory, what effects would this drug have?

A. Increase in inotropic and chronotropic effect.
B. Vasodilatation and bronchodilatation.
C. Vasoconstriction and bronchoconstriction.
D. Decrease in inotropic and chronotropic effect.

110. The primary neurotransmitter of the parasympathetic branch of the autonomic nervous system is:

   A. Acetylcholine.
   B. Succinylcholine.
   C. Norepinephrine.
   D. Dopamine.

111. Which of the following physiologic responses occur when the parasympathetic branch of the autonomic nervous system is stimulated?

   (1) Pupils dilate.
   (2) Heart rate decreases.
   (3) Peristalsis increases.
   (4) Sphincter tone increases.

   A. 1, 4.
   B. 2, 3.
   C. 2, 4.
   D. 1, 3.

112. You are treating a 21-year-old female who is in cardiovascular collapse secondary to a systemic reaction from a bee sting. She is in severe respiratory distress, and you have been unable to cannulate a vein or intubate her. Which of the following would be the best way to administer epinephrine to her?

   A. Intramuscular injection.
   B. Nebulized administration.
   C. Sublingual injection.
   D. Subcutaneous injection.

Answers with Rationale

1. (A) During ventricular relaxation and filling (diastole), the degree of vasoconstriction or dilatation present in the peripheral blood vessels (peripheral vascular resistance) determines the diastolic pressure. The difference between pressure during contraction (systole) and pressure during filling (diastole) is the pulse pressure.

2. (C) External rotation of the leg due to a fractured hip results in the movement of the leg away from the midline or midsagittal plane. This movement is termed abduction.

3. (C) An epiphyseal injury involves a fracture at the cartilaginous epiphysis, the growth center at the end of a long bone. Ginglymus describes a type of joint that allows movement in one plane only (e.g., the elbow). The diaphysis is the shaft of a long bone. The periosteum is a thick fibrous membrane that covers the surface of a bone.

4. (B) Nondescriptive terms such as "lethargic," "semi-comatose," and "somewhat confused" can be interpreted differently by different individuals. In order to give an accurate picture of how the patient is presenting in the field, you must report in objective terms what is taking place with the patient.

5. (B) The family history is rarely of immediate use in the field and is less important than the other information listed. Family history has little, if any, influence on the paramedic's assessment and management of an acute patient complaint and can be elicited during evaluation at the hospital. A history of allergies is always important and may alter present therapy. Knowledge of current medications assists in identifying underlying medical problems and may affect medication orders for this illness. Along with a history of the present illness, it is important to note any underlying medical problems such as cardiac, respiratory, or renal problems.

6. (C) Obtaining vital signs is part of the secondary survey and not part of the initial evaluation. Evaluation of circulation, hemorrhage, and level of consciousness should occur early during the primary survey to identify immediate, life-threatening problems.

7. (A) The "chief complaint" is the presenting symptom or the problem that prompted the call for help. The paramedic may respond to a traumatized victim and find a patient with obvious fractures who states "I can't breathe." In this situation the patient may have sustained other injuries, but the chief complaint is respiratory distress.

8. (A) Dilated pupils are caused by fright, pain, hypoxemia, brain injury, and ingestion of atropine-like drugs. Pupillary constriction is caused by CNS disorders, parasympathetic stimulation, ingestion of some narcotics, and proximity to a light source.

9. (C) Dysconjugate gaze occurs in head injury patients and is manifested by the failure of the eyes to function in a coordinated manner. Racoon's eyes is bilateral periorbital ecchymosis without evidence of direct injury. Doll's eyes is a lack of movement of the eyes when the head is turned quickly and is a normal sign. The doll's-eyes phenomenon may be lost when a brain injury has occurred, and the eyes may move toward the side where the head is turned. Battle's sign is a bluish discoloration over the tip of the mastoid bone.

10. (B) Partial loss of vision in both eyes occurs because the optic nerves from the two eyes meet at the optic chiasm, where some fibers cross over to the opposite side of the brain. The partial crossover provides both cerebral hemispheres with input from both eyes. Thus, the right occipital lobe controls the left lateral and right medial vision fields.

11. (D) Percussion is the eliciting of a tympanic note by striking body surfaces with the fingers. Inspection is observing the patient, auscultation is listening to the patient with a stethoscope, and palpation is feeling the patient.

12. (B) Pertinent negatives are statements by the patient denying symptoms that are important to the diagnosis.

13. (B) Nonrebreathing masks, when used correctly, will allow an FiO_2 of about 90%; simple masks allow about 50–60%, nasal cannulas 21–40%, and Venturi masks 24–50%.

14. (B) High airway pressures, commonly due to positive pressure/demand valves' short inspiratory time and valve malfunctions, often result in gastric distention/regurgitation. The valves also may rupture

weak spots in lung tissue, resulting in pneumothorax. The valves' drawbacks of weight, large oxygen consumption, and dependence on a power source are not as serious as their high airway pressures in terms of potential patient complications. Inability to evaluate lung compliance occurs but is less likely than excessive airway pressures.

15. (B) 800 cc is the minimum acceptable ventilation when resuscitating an adult, as recommended by the American Heart Association. Volume does not need to exceed 1200 cc.

16. (C) The head should be in the neutral position (if neck injury is suspected) or flexed during esophageal obturator airway (EOA) insertion. The sniff position or hyperextension should be avoided because of the possibility of tracheal placement.

17. (A) The esophageal obturator airway (EOA) is designed to reduce regurgitation of stomach contents. Once the EOA is placed, the rescuer must maintain correct patient head/neck position and keep a mask seal as with any bag-valve-mask device. Failure to do so is a common cause of inadequate EOA ventilation.

18. (D) Generally speaking, it is rare to achieve a larger ventilation with any device other than a pocket mask, whose ventilation depends on the rescuer's large expiratory volumes. The pocket mask is the preferred method of ventilation, according to the American Heart Association. Because of the pocket mask's simplicity, two hands can provide a seal and maintain the airway. At a 10 liters per minute O_2 flow, oxygen concentrations of 50% are usually delivered. If spontaneous respirations begin, the pocket mask may be used as a simple face mask.

19. (B) When initial attempts are unsuccessful, continue abdominal thrusts. As hypoxia worsens, the patient's muscles may relax and allow the object to be expelled. Blind finger sweeps should not be performed in the conscious patient. Transtracheal jet insufflation and pushing the object down the right bronchus are last resorts.

20. (A) Skin color changes in darkly pigmented people can best be observed in the mucous membranes of the mouth, the conjunctiva covering the sclera (white of the eye), or the nail beds.

21. (A) Direct pressure is the most effective technique for controlling bleeding. Pressure points are the second avenue of control and are used in conjunction with direct pressure or when it is impossible to reach the bleeding area. The application of a tourniquet is used only as a last resort. Potential hazards of tourniquets include damage to the blood vessels and nerves, and possible loss of an extremity.

22. (D) Abduction refers to movement away from the body. Flexion means forward movement, and extension means backward movement. Adduction refers to movement toward the body.

23. (A) The hamstring muscles behind the posterior thigh flex the knee. They are antagonists to the quadricep muscles in the anterior thigh. Most muscles work in a system that allows for opposite motions when one muscle provides a certain range of motion and an opposing muscle provides the opposite range of motion. Pronation and supination are also muscle functions, but they are not performed by the hamstring.

24. (C) Generally the nasogastric tube is measured from the tip of the nose to the earlobe, and then to the xiphoid process. After identifying the area on the tube, you should advance it to that point (approximately 20 inches). A fairly reliable indication of proper placement is rapid return of gastric contents when the tube is aspirated.

25. (A) The equipment needed for nasogastric tube insertion in a conscious patient includes a Levine tube, a 50-cc syringe, and a cup of water with a straw. A water-soluble lubricant should always be used instead of a lipid substance (Vasoline), which might be aspirated by the patient. The Levine tube is essential to the process, as is a large syringe to aspirate stomach contents. Tube insertion is much easier if the patient cooperates and is able to swallow water as the tube is passed.

26. (B) The EOA may be used in patients older than 16 years of age who are over five feet tall and who do not have known esophageal disease. If someone has an obstructed airway, blindly pushing the EOA into the pharynx may further lodge the object. EOA use should be avoided in patients who have bleeding into the pharynx. Obturation of the esophagus in these patients would cause fluid to follow the trachea.

27. (B) When using a straight blade, it is inserted under or posterior to the epiglottis. The epiglottis is directly lifted out of the way to expose the vocal cords.

28. (A) The first bifurcation of the trachea produces two bronchi. The right bronchus branches from the trachea more gradually than the longer left bronchus. Consequently, most objects (endotracheal tubes included) that are pushed down the trachea will lodge in the right main stem bronchus.

29. (B) Tracheal suction should never exceed 10 seconds. During normal suction, 4 liters of air will be removed from the lungs in 15 seconds. Limiting suction to 10 seconds or less and providing a high oxygen concentration before and after suctioning will prevent the most common complication, hypoxia. Suction pressure must be greater than 30 mm Hg in order to accomplish effective tracheal suction for the adult; pressures must be adjusted for infants and children. Continuous suction is maintained during catheter withdrawal to prevent secretions from being separated from the catheter. Failure to rotate the catheter may result in trauma to the tracheal mucosa.

30. (C) Bag-valve-mask units should not be equipped with pop-off valves because the pressures required for adequate ventilation may be greater than those which cause activation of the pop-off mechanism. The oxygen inlet and reservoir system, true nonrebreathing valve, and nonjam valve system have the ability to deliver an oxygen concentration of 100%.

31. (D) In order to align the axes of the mouth, pharynx, and trachea, the neck must be flexed forward and the head must be extended backward. This puts the head into a "sniffing" position. No other position overcomes anatomical angles and produces the straight line required for visualization of the vocal cords.

32. (B) Inadvertent intubation of the esophagus is among the hazards of endotracheal intubation. It is therefore necessary to auscultate the chest as soon as possible to verify pulmonary ventilation. Auscultation over the epigastrium provides another confirmation that the tube has been correctly placed. Although intubation of one bronchus generally involves the right mainstem bronchus because it is shorter and straighter than the left, both lungs must be auscultated to ensure that bilateral ventilation is being accomplished.

33. (A) The laryngeal skeleton is formed mostly by the cricoid cartilage (inferior portion) and the thyroid cartilage (superior portion). The top of the thyroid cartilage is attached to the hyoid bone by the thyrohyoid membrane. The vocal cords project from the arytenoid cartilage to the thyroid cartilage.

34. (D) The false vocal cords partially overlap and follow the course of the true vocal cords between the arytenoid and thyroid cartilages. False vocal cords are not as highly developed as true vocal cords and do not come together completely during normal voice production. They can close together and act as an important sphincter to protect the airway from aspiration of foreign material. When in spasm, the false vocal cords obscure the view of the true vocal cords and glottis from above.

35. (B) Use of the MacIntosh, or curved, blade requires placement of the blade into the vallecula located in the hypopharynx. The vallecula is the space between the base of the tongue and the epiglottis. The oropharynx extends from the soft palate to the epiglottis.

36. (B) The primary objective in securing an airway with an endotracheal tube is to prevent the aspiration of foreign material. Inflation of the cuff seals the lower airway and prevents aspiration of blood, stomach contents, or secretions.

37. (A) The PTLA is inserted into the patient's mouth until the bite block is in place between the patient's teeth. Once this is accomplished, both cuffs on the tube are inflated. The paramedic must then determine if the long tube has been placed in the trachea or in the esophagus since PTLA insertion is a blind technique. Nonproductive ventilation attempts in the short tube indicate that the long tube has been inserted into the trachea. The stylet is then removed and ventilations continued in the same manner as with an endotracheal tube.

38. (D) The PTLA device consists of two tubes with an internal diameter of 8 millimeters which lie side-by-side. One tube is 31 centimeters in length and the other is 21 centimeters. These lengths were selected to prevent the long tube from entering the right mainstem bronchus and the shorter tube from blocking the epiglottis. The long tube functions in the trachea as an endotracheal tube or in the esophagus as an obturator since it is equipped with a removable obturator stylet. The upper airway is sealed with a large balloon inflatable cuff in the mouth and pharynx,

eliminating the need for a mask. If the long tube is placed in the esophagus, ventilation is accomplished through the shorter tube. If no signs of ventilation are present, the long tube has been positioned in the trachea. In this situation, the obturator stylet is removed, and ventilation is provided through the longer tube.

39. (B) Vagal stimulation and hypoxia may cause bradyrhythmia to occur during endotracheal intubation attempts. Since the airway is patent, it is necessary to discontinue the intubation effort and hyperventilate the patient with 100% oxygen for 3 minutes. Once the patient has been properly oxygenated, intubation should be accomplished as quickly as possible.

40. (B) The Sellick maneuver is most frequently used to prevent regurgitation and aspiration of stomach contents. Compressing the larynx to perform a Sellick maneuver during some difficult intubations may alter the anatomy to make intubation easier.

41. (C) In order for you to perform a blind nasotracheal intubation, the patient must be breathing. The tube is advanced until there is air exchange through the ET tube. A relative contraindication is the possibility of a basilar skull fracture and disruption to the cribberform plate. The tube could contact brain tissue. This is a potential complication, but it is not frequently reported. It is regarded as a relative or possible contraindication. Nasotracheal intubation is appropriate in the responsive patient in respiratory failure. It is also a useful technique in the trauma patient with suspected cervical injury who is breathing, since it requires less manipulation of the neck than oral intubation.

42. (C) Nasotracheal intubation is ruled out because the patient is apneic. Orotracheal intubation using the trauma precautions is the method of choice. This involves applying a cervical collar and manual stabilization of the spine during laryngoscopy and tube placement. The EOA is a poor choice because it obturates the esophagus and forces blood and secretions into the respiratory tree. The PTLA could have the same result as the EOA. Endotracheal intubation is the gold standard of airway management.

43. (D) The narrowest portion of the adult trachea is at the vocal cords, and intubation requires a cuffed ET tube. In children, the narrowest

part is at the cricoid cartilage. When the tube is placed, it passes through this narrow section and makes a cuffed tube unnecessary for adequate ventilation.

44. (A) Percutaneous transtracheal jet insufflation is an emergency ventilation technique. To accomplish the required high-flow, high-pressure ventilation, you will need a catheter of at least 14 gauge and an oxygen cylinder with a hand-operated ON-OFF valve and reducing valve that yields 50 psi. A bag-valve-mask is not utilized in this procedure.

45. (B) Oxygen and nutrients are necessary for cellular function. If the heart is unable to pump blood adequately, blood/fluid volume is low, the vessels dilate, and blood cells are unable to carry oxygen and nutrients; thus shock occurs.

46. (A) A trauma patient found in shock without obvious signs of bleeding should be aggressively treated for hypovolemic (low blood volume) shock. The patient may be suffering from an undetected internal injury or hemorrhage.

47. (D) When the arterial pressure falls below 80 mm Hg, decreased blood flow occurs through the capillaries resulting in anaerobic metabolism, a change in capillary permeability, and an increase in red cell aggregation.

48. (C) Septic shock is usually caused by infectious states and results in the release of endotoxins from the gram-negative bacteria. Spinal cord injuries result in neurogenic shock. Internal hemorrhage leads to a hypovolemic shock state. Cardiogenic shock can occur when severe, life-threatening arrhythmias are persistent, or when a large area of the myocardium is damaged.

49. (A) Cardiogenic shock occurs when the heart is unable to be effective as a pump to meet the body's need for oxygen. Myocardial infarction is the most common cause of the heart's loss of effectiveness as a pump. The mortality rate from cardiogenic shock caused by myocardial infarction is high. Hypovolemic shock occurs when the body's total fluid volume is decreased. Neurogenic shock results when the reflex sympathetic response to decreased blood pressure is lost, and reflex peripheral vasoconstriction no longer occurs.

50. (C) Anaerobic metabolism occurs as a result of hypotension and hypoxia. Lactic acid production increases and cellular pH decreases. As lactic acid accumulates, precapillary arterioles relax, resulting in a decrease in capillary pressure. This leads to decreased capillary permeability, allowing blood to accumulate in the capillaries. This further decreases blood volume, leading to cellular death from insufficient oxygenation.

51. (A) When blood volume decreases, the amount of stretch placed on the baroreceptors decreases. This results in a stimulation of the sympathetic nervous system, causing an increased heart rate and an increase in peripheral vascular resistance, leading to sympathetic vasoconstriction. Peripheral vasoconstriction causes the skin to become cool and clammy.

52. (C) In third space fluid loss, plasma or extracellular fluid escapes into the interstitial spaces or a hollow body cavity. This fluid is no longer available for use by the circulatory system, even though it is not lost from the body. Pericardial tamponade results in cardiogenic shock. The physiological effects of cardiogenic shock are very similar to those of hypovolemic shock. Spinal cord injury, due to the interruption of fibers traveling from the brain stem's cardiovascular centers to the sympathetic centers in the spinal cord, leads to neurogenic shock.

53. (D) Tension pneumothorax results in a backflow of blood and jugular neck vein distention. Hypotension does not increase neck vein distention but, conversely, causes vessel collapse. A dissecting aneurysm causes decreased blood flow to the right side of the heart.

54. (B) A crystalloid solution such as lactated Ringer's or normal saline should be used in the initial fluid resuscitation of a patient in hypovolemic shock. This fluid causes intravascular expansion. It is a usual practice to administer three times the amount of crystalloid solution as blood lost.

55. (D) Anaphylactic shock occurs when an antigen interacts with an antibody in tissues that have been sensitized. This reaction causes the release of vasoactive amines that increase capillary permeability. Increased capillary permeability produces pulmonary edema, capillary vasodilation, and contraction of smooth muscles, causing bronchospasm and respiratory distress.

56. (A) When blood flow decreases through the kidneys, urinary output will decrease. At the same time, the renin-angiotensin mechanism is activated in an attempt to restore normal blood pressure. Due to this compensatory response, early signs of shock are sometimes not detected. Dehydration of cells results from fluid loss, but does not cause decreased urinary output.

57. (D) Sodium is the most abundant positive ion (cation) in the extracellular fluid and a major factor in maintaining osmotic pressure of the extracellular fluid.

58. (C) For every liter of isotonic fluid infused, about 1/4 actually stays in the vascular space and 3/4 leaks out. Although this leakage occurs slowly, it is an important factor when resuscitating patients with crystalloid solution. Crystalloids temporarily expand blood volume, but they do not carry oxygen. Therefore, patients must have a sufficient amount of blood to expand.

59. (B) A hypotonic solution causes cells to expand by osmosis. A hypertonic solution causes fluid to shift from within the cell to outside the cell. An isotonic solution causes no shift.

60. (A) Colloid solutions contain proteins which tend to keep them in the vascular space. Crystalloids tend to leak out. (Refer to Question 58.)

61. (B) Isotonic solutions have solute concentrations equal to that of the extracellular fluid and, therefore, do not change osmotic pressure.

62. (C) Blood volume is equal to 6–8% of ideal body weight. Blood weighs about 1 pound/pint.

63. (B) Normal pH is 7.4 with a range of 7.35 to 7.45. A solution with a pH of 1 would be a strong acid and 10 would be a strong base.

64. (B) The buffer system immediately absorbs hydrogen ions and produces carbonic acid. The respiratory system is activated within a few minutes and blows off the carbon dioxide. The kidneys are activated within hours to eliminate acids.

65. (C) Carbonic acid is a weak acid formed when hydrogen ions combine with bicarbonate. Acidotic patients frequently have increased respiratory rates because carbonic acid is eliminated mostly by the respiratory system.

66. (D) In hypovolemic states the body has a "pecking order" or a physiologic mechanism of "robbing Peter to pay Paul": skin, kidney, liver, heart/lungs, and brain. The skin is the first organ to be affected as a result of vasoconstriction due to sympathetic stimulation. The brain is the last organ to have blood shunted from it.

67. (C) When blood volume drops, the baroreceptors quickly sense the drop in pressure. They in turn notify the brain, which stimulates the sympathetic branch of the autonomic nervous system. Epinephrine and norepinephrine are released into the bloodstream to direct nerve stimulation of the heart and blood vessels, which results in increased heart rate and vasoconstriction in proportion to the blood loss. The net result is that the BP is maintained. Remaining alert for signs of this compensatory mechanism is crucial in the early recognition and management of blood loss.

68. (A) Falling blood pressure is a late indication of shock or bleeding. Long before the BP drops there are other obvious signs of compensation (tachycardia, pallor, delayed capillary refill, thirst, increased respiratory rate). When the BP begins to fall the patient usually has a 30% or greater blood loss and is in uncompensated shock.

69. (C) In a healthy patient a 30% blood loss can occur before compensation mechanisms fail and the blood pressure begins to fall.

70. (B) Neurogenic shock results from spinal cord injury and is caused by an interruption of the sympathetic outflow. Patients with head injuries and rising intracranial pressures have different vital signs than the patient in shock. Head injury produces a falling blood pressure as a terminal event.

71. (B) When the spinal cord is damaged, the autonomic nervous system does not stimulate vasoconstriction and increased heart rate as normal compensatory mechanisms. Messages cannot travel down a damaged cord. Therefore, the BP falls but the classic signs of compensation are absent. This is especially true with high spinal cord injuries.

72. (D) Patients with increasing intracranial pressure usually have rising blood pressure and falling pulse rate, due to decreased blood flow of the vasomotor center. Neurogenic shock is caused by the falling blood pressure that results from high spinal cord or brain stem injuries.

73. (A) One of the earliest post resuscitative complications of shock is adult respiratory distress syndrome (ARDS). Both renal and hepatic failure tend to be later complications.

74. (B) The tilt test is a useful test for nontraumatic hypovolemic patients, but it is not recommended for trauma patients. A heart rate increase of 20 beats or more per minute is considered a positive sign of hypovolemia. The tilt test is also considered positive if the patient becomes faint while being moved from supine to sitting.

75. (B) Short, large-bore IV catheters provide greater flow. To maximize flow during resuscitation, the length of the administration set tubing must be as short as possible.

76. (B) The patient has obvious signs of compensated shock and a narrow pulse pressure. Since his BP is >100 mm, he is not in progressive or decompensated shock at this time. Decompensated shock in an otherwise healthy trauma patient usually occurs after a greater than 25% or Grade III hemorrhage.

77. (B) While not an absolute rule, a trauma patient who has lost 20–25% of blood volume in 10 minutes is likely to appear moribund (unresponsive, no pulses, appears dead) within 20 minutes without intervention.

78. (D) While fluid therapy and PASG may gain this patient some time, he needs early surgical intervention. Fluid therapy and PASG should be attempted while en route to the nearest appropriate hospital. Intubation may be necessary later in the care of this patient, but it is not indicated at this point.

79. (A) Check carotid and femoral pulses when peripheral pulses are not palpable. If carotid and femoral pulses are present, systolic pressure is usually above 60 mm Hg.

80. (C) The initial fluid challenge recommended for a pediatric patient is 10–20 cc/kg.

81. (A) The use of vasopressor agents may be indicated in the prehospital treatment of neurogenic, cardiogenic, and anaphylactic shock in an effort to increase peripheral resistance or to increase myocardial contractility. When treating hypovolemic shock, it is of little value to increase vascular resistance or to increase myocardial contractility if the "tank" is empty of fluid.

82. (C) Metabolism of drugs occurs primarily in the liver. Normal doses of drugs may reach toxic levels in individuals with impaired liver function. For example, a patient with cirrhosis of the liver may develop signs of toxicity while receiving a lidocaine infusion that is well within the usual dosage range. Individuals with chronic obstructive pulmonary disease, gastroenteritis, and cholecystitis should not have significant alterations with biotransformation of drugs.

83. (A) The rate of absorption of medication from the fastest to the slowest route is: intravenous, endotracheal, sublingual, rectal, intramuscular, subcutaneous, and oral. One-half to two milliliters of solution may be administered subcutaneously. The needle angle is 45 degrees with a 5/8-inch-long 25-gauge needle. The skin is grasped and pulled away from underlying muscle during the injection.

84. (B) Synergism is the term used when drugs are combined and their effect is greater than the sum of their individual effects. A cumulative action results in an increased blood level following administration of several doses of a drug. Hypersensitivity results in an allergic-type reaction. Idiosyncrasy is an abnormal reaction to a drug.

85. (D) This solution requires a two-step calculation. First, the number of grains is converted to milligrams: 1 grain = 60 milligrams, thus 1/8 grain = 60 milligrams X 1/8 = 7.5 mg. Second, the volume needed to administer 7.5 mg is computed:

$$10 \text{ mg}/1 \text{ ml} = 7.5 \text{ mg}/ ? \text{ ml}$$
$$? = 7.5 \text{ mg X } 1 \text{ ml}/10 \text{ mg}$$
$$? = 0.75 \text{ ml}$$

86. (C) 200 cc/hour X 15 gtts/cc = 3000 gtts/hour
    3000 gtts ÷ 60 minutes = 50 gtts/minute

87. (D) The apothecary system of weights is the historical method of measurement based on common measures. The metric system was devised

to standardize an accurate measurement system and is used primarily for pharmacological measurement.

88. (C) The main purpose for pinching the IV tubing proximal to the injection site is to cause the medication to go into the vein rather than backing up into the IV tubing. In some cases, medications should not be allowed to mix with the IV solution (e.g., Valium) and should be injected right at the IV insertion site.

89. (A) When the thickness of subcutaneous tissue is diminished, the needle can penetrate the muscle tissue to a greater depth.

90. (B) The farmer could have absorbed, inhaled, and even ingested quantities of the insecticide, but injection would not occur under normal circumstances.

91. (D) You wish to establish a 4 mg/min lidocaine drip. One gram = 1000 milligrams (mg); 0.25 L = 250 milliliters (ml). The mg/ml concentration is determined by dividing 250 into 1000 which equals 4 mg/ml. Microdrop tubing has a drop factor of 60 gtts = 1 ml. Therefore, 60 gtts = 4 mg. Using the following formula:

$$\frac{\text{Desired dose}}{\text{Dose on hand}} \text{ X Vehicle} = \text{Volume Administered}$$

The solution would be:

$$\frac{4 \text{ mg/min}}{4 \text{ mg/ml}} \text{ X } \frac{60 \text{ gtts/ml}}{1} \text{ X } \frac{240 \text{ gtts/min}}{4} = 60 \text{ gtts/min}$$

92. (A) Changes of the gastrointestinal system produced by food, emotion, and physical activity make the oral route of drug administration the most unreliable and slowest. These changes affect both the amount and the rate of drug absorption. Although sublingual administration depends on the patient's ability to cooperate, medications are quickly absorbed via this route. Parenteral routes, such as subcutaneous, afford relatively rapid drug absorption since the epithelial barriers are avoided. The intravenous route of administration completely bypasses the process of absorption and is the most rapid means of introducing drugs into the body.

93. (D) Tinctures are prepared by extracting the drug chemically, usually with alcohol (e.g., tincture of iodine). Lotions are usually aqueous prepa-

rations containing suspended material and are used as cleansing agents or astringents. Astringents possess a "drawing" action. Elixirs are preparations that contain the medicinal agent in an alcohol solvent. Artificial flavoring is usually added to enhance the flavor. Suppositories contain medication that has been mixed into a base which is solid at room temperature but dissolves at body temperature. Medication in suppositories is absorbed rectally or vaginally. Spirits contain volatile chemicals dissolved in alcohol. When exposed to room air, these mixtures evaporate rapidly (e.g., spirits of ammonia) and are inhaled by the patient.

94. (C) Suspensions are medications that do not remain dissolved in the solvent. Since the solid material separates from the liquid, the container must be shaken well prior to administration.

95. (B) In order to absorb medications that are administered via intramuscular (IM) or subcutaneous (SQ) routes, the patient must have adequate tissue perfusion. A patient who is cold, clammy, and pale is suspect of inadequate tissue perfusion and, therefore, would not be a candidate for either IM or SQ routes of administration. These patients would require intravenous drug administrations.

96. (A) When increasingly higher dosages of a medication are required to achieve the same therapeutic effect, the patient has developed a tolerance to the drug. Habituation implies a physical or psychological drug dependency. When the drug produces a side effect that is harmful to the patient, this is identified as an untoward effect. A cumulative action occurs when several doses of a drug are administered, causing an increased effect. This usually results from a quantitative intravascular accumulation of the drug.

97. (C) This patient is experiencing a common side effect of sulfa drugs. An allergic reaction (hypersensitivity) includes signs and symptoms associated with the release of histamine (e.g., urticaria, itching, wheezing, etc.). Potentiation involves the enhancement of one drug by another. Synergism is the joint action of drugs such that their combined effect is greater than the sum of their individual effects.

98. (D) When medical or physiological conditions are present in a patient that would make it harmful to administer a medication of otherwise known therapeutic value, it is considered to be contraindicated. It is

possible that the physician did not hear the entire radio transmission and ordered pharmacological intervention based on the partial information received. It is also possible that the paramedic did not communicate all pertinent information prior to requesting orders. Therefore, the paramedic should question the order by supplying the information that demonstrates the medication is contraindicated. In any event, the paramedic should always repeat orders before initiating them.

99. (A) Each tablet contains 0.5 grams or 500 mg. Using the following formula:

$$\frac{\text{Desired dose}}{\text{Dose on hand}} \times \text{Vehicle} = \text{Amount to be administered}$$

The solution is:

$$\frac{750 \text{ mg}}{500 \text{ mg/tablet}} \times \frac{1 \text{ tablet}}{1} = \frac{750 \text{ mg}}{500 \text{ mg}} = 1.5 \text{ tablets}$$

100. (A) Determine how many mg/ml you have available. 0.5 mg = 1000 (milligrams in 1 gram) = 500 mg. 0.02 L $\times$ 1000 (milliliters in 1 liter) = 20.

$$\frac{\text{Desired dose}}{\text{Dose on hand}} \times \text{Vehicle} = \text{Volume administered}$$

$$\text{Dose on hand} = \frac{500 \text{ mg}}{20 \text{ ml}} = 25 \text{ mg/ml}$$

The solution is:

$$\frac{150 \text{ mg}}{25 \text{ mg/ml}} \times \frac{1 \text{ ml}}{1} = \frac{150}{25} = 6 \text{ ml}$$

101. (A) In order to determine the number of drops that must be administered per minute in order to infuse the medication as ordered, you must apply the following formula:

$$\frac{\text{Total volume (in milliliters)}}{\text{Total time (in minutes)}} \times \frac{\text{Drops per ml}}{1} = \text{\# Drops per minute}$$

The solution is as follows:

$$\frac{100}{20} \times \frac{10}{1} = \frac{1000}{20} = 50 \text{ gtts/min}$$

102. (B) Using the following formula:

$$\frac{\text{Desired dose}}{\text{Dose on hand}} \times \text{Vehicle} = \text{Volume administered}$$

The solution is:

$$\frac{30}{15} \times \frac{0.50}{1} = \frac{15.0}{15.0} = 1.00 \text{ ml}$$

103. (C) Since the total dosage is dependent on the patient's body weight, you must first convert pounds to kilograms. This is accomplished by dividing 2.2 (2.2 pounds per kg) into 165 pounds, which equals 75 kg. The patient is to receive 0.01 mg for every kg (0.01 X 75) or a total of 0.75 mg. A 1:1000 solution contains 1 mg in 1 ml. Using the following formula:

$$\frac{\text{Desired dose}}{\text{Dose on hand}} \times \text{Vehicle} = \text{Volume administered}$$

The solution is:

$$\frac{0.75}{1.00} \times \frac{1.00}{1} = \frac{0.75}{1.00} = 0.75 \text{ ml}$$

104. (B) Following orders immediately after receiving them over the radio increases the possibility of medication errors. The paramedic must always repeat orders after they are transmitted to help prevent misunderstanding and to confirm that what the paramedic heard was what Medical Control actually ordered.

105. (A) The needle used for a subcutaneous injection is usually 24, 25, or 26 gauge. The larger the number the smaller the diameter of the needle. The required length varies from 3/8 inch to 1 inch, depending upon the size and hydration of the patient. A longer needle is needed for an obese patient, a shorter needle for a dehydrated person. Generally, a 25-gauge needle, 5/8 inch in length is used for an average adult.

106. (D) Intramuscular (IM) injection is the method of choice for the administration of some medications. Drugs that irritate subcutaneous (SQ) tissue are often given IM. In addition, a larger amount of fluid can be delivered into the muscle than into SQ tissue. Absorption through the

muscle is faster than absorption through SQ tissue due to the vascularity of the muscle area. However, the danger of damaging nerves and blood vessels is greater with IM injections.

107. (B) A useful mnemonic to remember which drugs can be administered via an ET tube is NALE: Naloxone Atropine Lidocaine Epinephrine. Other drugs either irritate the lung tissue or are not easily absorbed. Although diazepam has been absorbed through bronchial trees of animals, it has not been approved for ET tube administration in humans.

108. (B) In order to ensure adequate distribution and absorption through the bronchial tree, it is recommended that the drug be administered in 10 cc of solution.

109. (B) Beta-2 effects on the autonomic nervous system include bronchodilatation and vasodilatation. Increased inotropic and chronotropic effects are Beta-1. Bronchoconstriction and vasoconstriction are Alpha effects.

110. (A) The neurotransmitter of the parasympathetic system is acetylcholine. Succinylcholine is a paralytic agent and dopamine is a vasopressor. Norepinephrine is a sympathetic neurotransmitter.

111. (B) When the parasympathetic branch is stimulated the heart rate decreases and an increase in peristaltic movement occurs. Dilated pupils and increased sphincter tone are results of sympathetic stimulation.

112. (C) The sublingual area is a rich vascular bed capable of rapid absorption even in low perfusion states. While rarely used, this is an acceptable site of medication delivery in extreme situations when other routes are not possible. If the epinephrine is administered by the subcutaneous or intramuscular route, it will not be absorbed until peripheral perfusion is restored. Nebulized epinephrine may not reach central circulation.

4 Trauma

Trauma
Burns

Trauma

1. A closed or simple fracture is best defined as a:

   A. Fracture in which the overlying skin is intact.
   B. Fracture of a long bone with skin discoloration over the affected area.
   C. Fracture with associated ligament involvement.
   D. Fracture with associated muscle spasms or swelling around a joint.

2. Which of the following statements is *not* true concerning sprains?

   A. Splinting is not necessary with sprains.
   B. A sprain involves injury to the ligaments.
   C. Treatment of a sprain includes elevation of the joint and application of cold packs.
   D. Signs and symptoms of a sprain include pain, ecchymosis, and swelling.

3. When assessing a fracture, the paramedic must first:

   A. Assess the proximal pulses to evaluate arterial status.
   B. Correct any angulation so that the pain is reduced.
   C. Apply the appropriate splint.
   D. Evaluate the circulatory status distal to the injury.

4. You are called to the local ice skating rink where a 16-year-old boy has fallen and injured his left arm. During your assessment, you notice swelling and deformity of the left forearm, and the boy complains of tenderness when touched. The pulse is strong, and there is no loss of sensation in the fingers. You apply and carefully inflate an air splint. While you are en route to the hospital, the young man complains of a "pins and needles" sensation in his left hand. You would immediately:

   A. Remove the splint and allow the arm to hang dependent to improve blood flow.
   B. Slightly deflate the air splint.
   C. Carefully massage the arm, in order to stimulate circulation, after removal of the splint.
   D. Realize that paresthesia is to be expected after a fracture and explain this to the boy.

5. A 17-year-old football player fell on his shoulder during practice. You suspect a fractured clavicle and treat him by applying a:

    A. Sling and swathe.
    B. Pillow splint.
    C. Traction splint.
    D. Rigid splint.

6. A 39-year-old female was injured while working at the local book bindery. She complains of considerable pain to her right shoulder, with loss of motion. While comparing the right and left shoulders, you notice an anterior bulge of the right shoulder. You suspect she is suffering from a(n):

    A. Fracture of the humeral head.
    B. Dislocation of the femoral neck.
    C. Anterior shoulder dislocation.
    D. Strain to the trapezius muscle.

7. Your 12-year-old patient fell out of his tree house. His left arm is bent across his chest, and he complains of a great deal of pain. You suspect a fractured left elbow. Appropriate care would include:

    A. Evaluation of distal pulses and the application of a sling and swathe.
    B. Evaluation of distal pulses and the application of a rigid splint to the left arm.
    C. Evaluation of proximal pulses and the application of a rigid splint to the left arm.
    D. Evaluation of proximal pulses and the application of a padded board splint to the left arm.

8. Your patient is a 16-year-old boy who lost control of his motorcycle. Examination reveals angulation of the right lower leg. During your evaluation of the patient you wish to assess the posterior tibial pulse. You know that this pulse is found:

    A. Behind the knee.
    B. In front of the medial malleolus.
    C. Behind the medial malleolus.
    D. On the dorsum of the foot.

9. Joints are important structures because they allow for skeletal mobility. Which of the following structures are most important in providing support for these relatively unstable structures?

A. Fascia.
B. Muscles.
C. Ligaments.
D. Joint capsule.

10. Which of the following statements is most correct concerning open fractures?

A. An open fracture is one in which a portion of bone protrudes through the skin.
B. A bullet may cause an open fracture.
C. Open fractures must be reduced prior to splinting.
D. An open fracture is also known as a comminuted fracture.

11. Which of the following is the *least* common sign or symptom of musculoskeletal injury?

A. Pain.
B. Inability to move an extremity or joint.
C. Swelling.
D. Deformity.

12. A closed fracture of which of the following may produce the largest blood loss?

A. Humerus.
B. Tibia-fibula.
C. Femur.
D. Pelvis.

13. Peter Lucas is an unconscious patient who has been involved in a vehicular accident. Your assessment reveals the following: decreased level of consciousness; left pupil dilated and nonreactive to direct light; pulse 70, full and bounding; respirations 16/min; BP 124/70. Assuming that intracranial pressure continues to increase, you would anticipate which of the following changes in Peter's blood pressure and pulse:

A. Narrowing pulse pressure, bradycardia.
B. Widening pulse pressure, tachycardia.

    C. Narrowing pulse pressure, tachycardia.
    D. Widening pulse pressure, bradycardia.

14. While assessing a head-injured patient with increased pressure on the reticular activating system and the left oculomotor nerve, you would most likely observe:

    A. Hyperirritability, dilation of the left pupil.
    B. Hyperirritability, constriction of the left pupil.
    C. Decreased level of consciousness, dilation of the left pupil.
    D. Decreased level of consciousness, constriction of the left pupil.

15. Which of the following breathing patterns is not likely to be exhibited by the brain-injured patient?

    A. Cheyne-Stokes respirations.
    B. Kussmaul breathing.
    C. Central neurogenic hyperventilation.
    D. Apnea.

16. Which of the following positions would *least* likely be assumed by a patient with a spinal cord injury?

    A. Forearms flexed across chest.
    B. Extension of legs and flexion of arms.
    C. Hands held above head.
    D. Head tilted to one side.

17. Patients with head injuries should also routinely be treated for which of the following conditions?

    A. Blood loss.
    B. Respiratory depression.
    C. Spinal cord injury.
    D. Cardiac arrhythmias.

Questions 18–20 relate to the following situation:

You are dispatched to a high school softball diamond where a player has been struck by a softball in the left temporal area. When you arrive on the scene, you find a 17-year-old female who is alert and oriented to person, time, and place. She is complaining of pain in the left temporal area, and you observe bruising and elicit complaints of pain upon palpation. The coach tells you the patient was unconscious immediately after the blow and was out for four to five minutes. She regained consciousness about one minute before your arrival. The rest of the history and physical exam are noncontributory. En route to the hospital, the patient's LOC begins to deteriorate, and she lapses into coma.

18. Following an assessment, you suspect that this patient has which of the following conditions?

    A. Subdural hematoma.
    B. Brain laceration.
    C. Epidural bleeding.
    D. Concussion.

19. The patient's rapid deterioration and location of injury suggest:

    A. An injury to the area of the brain that controls consciousness.
    B. An arterial bleed.
    C. Hidden bleeding elsewhere in the body.
    D. Contusion of the brain.

20. You suspect she does not have a basilar skull fracture due to the absence of:

    A. Periorbital ecchymosis and bruising behind the ear.
    B. Periorbital ecchymosis and doll's eyes.
    C. Watery drainage from the ears and a Babinski response.
    D. Watery drainage from the ears and respiratory depression.

21. The hematoma/hemorrhage that is most often masked by the presence of alcohol in the patient's body, is a(n):

    A. Epidural hematoma.
    B. Subarachnoid hemorrhage.
    C. Subdural hematoma.
    D. Intracerebral hemorrhage.

22. Spinal injuries occur most frequently to which of the following vertebrae?

    A. Cervical and thoracic.
    B. Thoracic and lumbar.
    C. Cervical and lumbar.
    D. Thoracic and sacral.

23. Which statement best characterizes pressure on the spinal cord?

   A. It always leads to permanent loss of function.
   B. It may be the result of bone fragments or a displaced disc.
   C. It is always associated with severe pain at the site of the injury.
   D. It requires no special field management.

24. Hypoventilation occurs in the spinal cord-injured patient as a result of:

   A. Patient guarding due to pain on inspiration.
   B. Damage to nerve fibers supplying the lungs.
   C. Damage to nerve fibers supplying the diaphragm.
   D. Hidden injuries elsewhere.

25. Heat loss occurs in the spinal cord-injured patient as a result of:

   A. Widespread peripheral vasodilation.
   B. Damage to heat-monitoring sensors.
   C. Loss of nerve supply to skeletal muscles.
   D. Reflex response of the hypothalamus.

26. Which of the following measures is considered standard treatment protocol for an unconscious patient with unknown etiology?

   A. Oxygen, Narcan, syrup of ipecac, spinal immobilization.
   B. Oxygen, dextrose, nitroglycerin, spinal immobilization.
   C. Oxygen, Narcan, dextrose, spinal immobilization.
   D. Oxygen, syrup of ipecac, Benadryl, spinal immobilization.

27. You are called to the scene of a swimming pool and find a 20-year-old male, who had been diving and had struck his head on the bottom of the pool. Your initial reaction is to:

   A. Complete a neurological examination.
   B. Manage him as if he sustained a spinal cord injury.
   C. Prepare to intubate him.
   D. Start an IV using a dextrose solution.

28. Which of the following statements is correct concerning spinal immobilization?

   A. The paramedic should apply manual stabilization.
   B. A C-collar is sufficient if the patient is cooperative.
   C. The torso should be immobilized as well as the neck.
   D. Immobilization is unnecessary if the patient has been walking around.

29. Following head trauma, a patient may exhibit hyperpnea and tachypnea. The pattern of respirations in which these are present is known as:

    A. Cheyne-Stokes respirations.
    B. Eupneic ventilation.
    C. Kussmaul respirations.
    D. Central neurogenic hyperventilation.

30. A 39-year-old male has been involved in a vehicular accident. Upon examination you note Battle's sign and blood flowing from the right ear. No other signs or injuries are visible. Vital signs are pulse 160 and thready, respirations 32 and shallow, and blood pressure 80 systolic by palpation. You suspect:

    A. Internal hemorrhage and head injury.
    B. Isolated head injury.
    C. Isolated internal hemorrhage.
    D. No major injuries.

31. Typically, a self-inflicted shotgun wound to the face presents a major airway maintenance problem. Select the adjunct most likely to secure the airway of such a patient.

    A. Nasopharyngeal airway.
    B. Endotracheal tube airway.
    C. Esophageal obturator airway.
    D. Oropharyngeal airway.

32. A patient with severe bleeding from the large vessels of the neck should:

    A. Be placed in a sitting position.
    B. Have direct pressure applied to the artery above the laceration.
    C. Have direct pressure applied to the veins above and below the laceration.
    D. Have a circumferential bandage applied to hold a pressure dressing in place.

33. You respond to a call where you find a 42-year-old female with a knitting needle impaled through her right cheek. Your assessment reveals active bleeding. You would:

    A. Stabilize the tip of the knitting needle in place with a bulky dressing and transport immediately.

    B. Remove the knitting needle in the same direction it entered and dress the wound inside the mouth and on the cheek.

    C. Remove the knitting needle in the opposite direction it entered, dress the entrance wound, and transport.

    D. Remove the knitting needle in the same direction it entered, apply a sterile dressing to the external wound, and transport.

34. Your first action in the management of open, soft tissue wounds should be to:

    A. Prevent further contamination.
    B. Control bleeding.
    C. Immobilize the injured area.
    D. Apply ice to the wound.

35. Amputated tissue can best be cared for by:

    A. Immersion in saline solution.
    B. Freezing.
    C. Wrapping in sterile dressing and cooling.
    D. Wrapping in sterile dressing and warming.

36. General management of a patient with an abdominal evisceration would include:

    A. Covering the area with a sterile dry dressing and taping it securely in place.

    B. Applying sterile saline dressings over the viscera and covering it with a bulky dry dressing.

    C. Applying a dry dressing over the wound and securing it with an abdominal binder.

    D. Replacing the organs and covering the area with a dressing soaked in saline solution.

37. The patient is a 19-year-old male who has sustained trauma to the upper left quadrant of the abdomen. He is conscious and complains of generalized abdominal pain. Vital signs are pulse 134 and weak; respirations 28, shallow and labored; blood pressure 96/40. Your care for this patient would include:

A. Oxygen per nasal cannula, IV lactated Ringer's TKO, supine position, cardiac monitor, and vital signs every 15 minutes.
B. Oxygen per mask, IV lactated Ringer's wide open, supine position with lower extremities slightly elevated, cardiac monitor, and vital signs every 15 minutes.
C. Oxygen per mask, IV D₅W to run 100 gtts per minute, supine position, cardiac monitor, and vital signs every 5 minutes.
D. Oxygen per nasal cannula, IV D₅W TKO, Trendelenburg's position, monitoring the electrocardiogram, and vital signs every 10–15 minutes.

38. Which of the following is a true statement concerning electrical burns?

A. Direct current is the most dangerous type of current.
B. Low-voltage electricity generates extreme heat in the body and follows the path of the blood vessels and nerves.
C. The least serious complications of electrical burns are internal injuries.
D. Electrical burns always produce extensive external burns.

39. A 21-year-old female suffered blunt trauma when her car crashed into a concrete abutment. Which of the following factors has the greatest influence in determining the kinetic energy involved in the collision?

A. Weight/mass of the patient.
B. Speed of the automobile.
C. Size of the automobile.
D. Size of the abutment.

40. An unrestrained occupant was ejected from a vehicle involved in a collision. An ejected occupant is _____ times more likely to die than an occupant who stays with the vehicle.

A. 2.
B. 4.
C. 6.
D. 8.

41. Given consistency of body tissue, direction of penetration, and range of weapon, which of the following causes the greatest tissue damage?

A. .44 Magnum pistol.
B. Bowie knife.
C. .357 Magnum pistol.
D. M-14 military rifle.

42. A 30-year-old prowler fell a distance of 20 feet and landed on his feet, breaking both ankles. The kinetics of this injury pattern are most commonly associated with which type of injury?

A. Spinal compression fracture.
B. C-1 and C-2 "hangman's" fracture.
C. Aortic tear from the ligamenta arteriosum.
D. Liver injury from the ligament of "teres."

Questions 43–46 relate to the following situation:

You are called to a multi-vehicle accident and arrive first on scene. There are a total of 12 patients, with back-up units 10–15 minutes away. You and your partner establish EMS command and begin the initial round of triage.

43. Your first patient is a 25-year-old male with altered mental status, an open chest wound, and bilateral femur fractures. You note that respirations are 30, radial pulse is not palpable, but the carotid pulse is present. You should triage this patient:

A. Priority 1 (Immediate/Red).
B. Priority 2 (Delayed/Yellow).
C. Priority 3 (Hold/Green).
D. Priority 0 (Dead/Black).

44. The second patient is a 30-year-old male who is unresponsive. He has massive head and maxillofacial injuries, and is breathing agonally after his airway is cleared. Pulse is slow and barely palpable, and there is massive bleeding into the oropharynx. You should triage this patient:

A. Priority 1 (Immediate/Red).
B. Priority 2 (Delayed/Yellow).
C. Priority 3 (Hold/Green).
D. Priority 0 (Dead/Black).

45. The third patient, a 12-year-old child, was ejected from the vehicle and is ambulatory. He complains of thirst and some nonspecific abdominal pain. He has a pulse of 120. You should triage this patient:

    A. Priority 1 (Immediate/Red).
    B. Priority 2 (Delayed/Yellow).
    C. Priority 3 (Hold/Green).
    D. Priority 0 (Dead/Black).

46. The fourth patient is a 20-year-old female who complains of cervical spine pain and is not oriented to person, place, or time. Radial pulses are easily palpable, and she seems to be moving an adequate amount of air. You should triage this patient:

    A. Priority 1 (Immediate/Red).
    B. Priority 2 (Delayed/Yellow).
    C. Priority 3 (Hold/Green).
    D. Priority 0 (Dead/Black).

47. You are treating a man who suffered blunt chest trauma and is dyspneic. Which of the following signs is of the *least* value in the early recognition of tension pneumothorax?

    A. Tracheal deviation.
    B. Tachycardia.
    C. Tachypnea.
    D. Unilateral absent breath sounds.

48. What is a key anatomic landmark when attempting to locate the second or third intercostal space in the midclavicular line for thoracic decompression?

    A. Hypothenar eminence.
    B. Angle of Louis.
    C. Point of maximal impulse.
    D. The xiphoid process.

Questions 49–51 relate to the following situation:

You are treating a 40-year-old male who suffered blunt trauma to the chest from a steering wheel injury. He complains of dyspnea and pleuritic chest pain. He was an *unrestrained occupant and has an obvious steering wheel pattern on the anterior chest. Physical exam reveals equal, clear breath sounds bilaterally, pulse 100, respirations 36, BP 146/88. ECG is sinus rhythm with an obvious bundle branch block and frequent ventricular ectopy. Pulse oximeter shows an adequate waveform and SpO$_2$ of 92. Rib cage appears to be intact with no obvious fractures or crepitus.*

49. What is your initial presumptive diagnosis?

    A. Pericardial tamponade.
    B. Pulmonary embolism.
    C. Acute myocardial infarction.
    D. Pulmonary contusion.

50. The bundle branch block and ectopy noticed on the ECG is most likely attributable to which of the following?

    (1) Pulmonary embolism.
    (2) Hypoxia.
    (3) Myocardial infarction.
    (4) Myocardial contusion.

    A. 1, 2.
    B. 2, 3.
    C. 3, 4.
    D. 2, 4.

51. Which of the following treatment modalities is *least* indicated in the prehospital management of this patient at this time?

    A. Antidysrhythmic therapy.
    B. High-concentration oxygen.
    C. Crystalloid volume challenge.
    D. Continued SpO$_2$ monitoring.

52. You are treating a 19-year-old male who has a stab wound to the upper left abdominal quadrant. Which of the following is *least* important in the initial management of this patient?

    A. Sealing the wound with an occlusive dressing.
    B. Establishing IV lines for volume replacement.
    C. Administration of high-concentration oxygen.
    D. Monitoring the electrocardiogram.

53. You are treating a 30-year-old patient who has sustained blunt trauma to the upper left abdominal quadrant and is being treated as a rule out spleen injury. Splenic injuries may cause pain to be referred to which of the following areas?

    A. Groin on the same side as the injury.
    B. Left shoulder.
    C. The umbilicus.
    D. Lumbar spine.

54. You are assessing an unconscious trauma patient who has a nondistended, soft abdomen. Which statement most accurately describes the reliability of this finding?

    A. Lack of distension and guarding rule out occult bleeding.
    B. Lack of distension and guarding does not rule out occult bleeding.
    C. Any significant bleeding is heralded by obvious distension.
    D. Any significant bleeding is heralded by involuntary guarding.

55. Which of the following is of *least* significance in the prehospital assessment of blunt or penetrating trauma to the abdomen?

    A. Monitoring of SpO_2.
    B. Auscultation of bowel sounds.
    C. Inspection of the abdomen.
    D. Palpation of the abdomen.

56. You are assessing a 10-year-old child who received blunt trauma to the chest and abdomen. Physical examination reveals crepitus and two obvious rib fractures on the right side. Which of the following statements is most correct?

    A. Rib fractures are not serious unless they puncture the pleura.
    B. The child is at high risk for significant internal injury.
    C. Rib fractures are common in children and are only serious in the elderly.
    D. Rib fractures should be treated by a snug restrictive bandage.

Burns

57. A 17-year-old high school senior has accidentally splashed sulfuric acid in his left eye during a chemistry lab. His lab partner tells you he is wearing contact lenses. His initial care would include:

A. Removal of contact lenses, flushing with large amounts of water, and patching both eyes.
B. Flushing with copious amounts of vinegar water and patching both eyes.
C. Removal of contact lenses, flushing with one part alcohol to three parts water, and patching the left eye.
D. Removal of contact lenses, flushing with baking soda water, and patching the left eye.

58. Twenty-one-year-old Rose has received burns on the front of both legs and on the front and back of both arms. Estimate the percentage of skin surface area that has been burned.

   A. 27%.
   B. 36%.
   C. 45%.
   D. 54%.

59. A severely burned patient should:

   A. Have debris picked off the skin.
   B. Be given 500–1000 ml of IV fluid per hour.
   C. Receive low-concentration O_2.
   D. Have all jewelry removed.

60. A first-degree burn is typically distinguished by:

   A. A painful, blistered area involving the epidermis.
   B. Pain and redness involving the epidermis.
   C. Painless brown or charred areas with areas of pallor.
   D. A painful area with blisters and pallor.

61. A burn lesion resembling a bull's-eye with blisters and with a charred central zone of third-degree burn, a middle zone of cold, gray second-degree burn, and an outer ring of red tissue is typical of a/an:

   A. Contact burn.
   B. Flash burn.
   C. Arc burn.
   D. Flame burn.

62. Three-year-old Cameron pulled a pot of boiling water off the stove and received second-degree burns on his head and neck, both arms, and his

entire (front and back) torso. What percentage of skin surface area has Cameron burned?

A. 45%.
B. 54%.
C. 72%.
D. 82%.

63. You respond to a call from the fire department for medical help at a three-alarm fire that is raging out of control. You and your partner are the first medical team to arrive at the scene; therefore, you need to identify the most critical patients and start treatment. Which of the following patients would receive your attention last, because the burn is not considered critical?

A. A patient with a 9% burn that includes both hands.
B. A patient with an 18%, superficial, second-degree burn over the body.
C. A patient with a 9%, superficial, second-degree burn of a fractured right arm.
D. A patient who is diabetic and has a 15%, deep, second-degree burn.

64. You are called to a local factory where a 26-year-old male has been sprayed with dry lime. All of the following instructions would be considered correct management for this patient except:

A. Brushing away all possible particles from the patient's body.
B. Covering any burned areas with sterile dressings.
C. Flushing the affected area for 5 to 10 minutes with water.
D. Removing jewelry and clothing from the patient.

65. You are called to a hardware store where Mr. Banks was involved in a furnace explosion. You note second-degree burns to his entire head and neck, anterior chest, anterior left leg, and entire left and right arms. Vital signs are P 120 and thready, R 30 and labored, BP 90/60. He is conscious and crying out in pain. Using the rule of nines, you would estimate the percentage of Mr. Banks' burns as:

A. 54%.
B. 45%.
C. 40.5%.
D. 36%.

66. Mr. Banks has no known allergies and weighs approximately 175 pounds. Using the Parkland Formula for fluid replacement and an IV tubing that delivers 10 gtts/ml, you would regulate the infusion of crystalloid fluid at:

    A. 100 gtts/min.
    B. 150 gtts/min.
    C. 200 gtts/min.
    D. 250 gtts/min.

67. During a heavy thunderstorm, a power line was broken by falling tree limbs. While attempting to secure the scene, a utility company worker came in contact with the live wire. When managing this situation, the paramedic must remember which principle?

    A. Electricity follows a path of least resistance.
    B. The least serious electrical burns are internal.
    C. AC current is the least dangerous form of electricity.
    D. Electricity typically produces devastating external burns.

68. Assessment of a 40-year-old female involved in a house fire reveals the patient sustained 30% BSA of second- and third-degree burns. Although the patient is conscious and crying out in pain, she is restless and dyspneic. All of the following would be included in the prehospital management of this patient except:

    A. Blind nasotracheal intubation.
    B. Analgesia with morphine sulfate or nitrous oxide.
    C. Wet sterile saline dressings to the injuries.
    D. Assisted ventilations with 100% oxygen.

69. Normal tissue perfusion requires a balance of the capillary and tissue pressures. All of the following exert a pulling force from the intravascular space in a direction to the interstitial space except:

    A. Capillary fluid pressure.
    B. Interstitial fluid pressure.
    C. Plasma colloid pressure.
    D. Interstitial colloid pressure.

70. Eric is a 15-year-old who was attempting to light a charcoal bed when his clothing ignited. Upon arrival, you find that the fire has been extin-

guished. The primary assessment is within normal limits. There are extensive second-degree burns on his trunk and both thighs. In transit to the hospital, you note the rapid development of edema in the areas of the burns. What is the physiological basis for this development?

A. Decrease in the overall intravascular peripheral resistance.
B. Shift in the plasma colloid osmotic pressure to the interstitium.
C. Rapid diffusion of fluids into the areas of injury as a natural response to tissue damage.
D. Decrease in the interstitial fluid pressure due to the vascular damage associated with burn injuries.

71. You are transporting a 40-year-old female weighing approximately 150 pounds who was extricated from her burning bedroom. Her pulse is 140, respirations are 32 and shallow, and her BP is 104/58. An IV of crystalloid fluid was established. Sterile dressings have been applied to the second- and third-degree burns she sustained on her anterior chest, anterior thighs, and right lateral aspect of her head. Oxygen administration was initiated immediately and has been continuous throughout. The estimated time of arrival (ETA) to the hospital is 30 minutes. The major life-threatening complication for this patient en route to the hospital would be:

A. Cardiac arrest, secondary to smoke inhalation.
B. Hypovolemic shock, secondary to fluid loss in the burns.
C. Airway obstruction, secondary to laryngeal edema.
D. Wound contamination, secondary to circumstances at the scene.

Answers with Rationale

1. (A) Closed or simple fractures are defined as fractures where the overlying skin is intact. An open or compound fracture occurs when there is a wound over the fracture site.

2. (A) Sprains are usually treated in the same manner as a fracture. Splinting of the sprain, in order to give support and prevent further damage, would be required.

3. (D) Assessment of distal pulses must be done in order to evaluate the circulatory status of the affected part. Pulses are checked before the correction of any angulation or application of a splint. If proximal pulses are assessed, as opposed to distal pulses, a problem farther down an extremity could be missed. For example, it is possible to have an intact brachial pulse and absent radial pulse with a fracture of an upper extremity.

4. (B) You must slightly deflate the air splint. When the splint is applied in a cold environment and moved into a warmer area, such as the ambulance, the splint tends to expand, leading to occlusion of blood flow to the extremity.

5. (A) The sling, with the addition of the swathe, provides immobilization of the fractured clavicle. A pillow splint is used to immobilize an injured foot or ankle. Traction splints are used when a constant pull on the injured lower extremity is needed. A rigid splint is a nonflexible device attached to a limb in order to immobilize it.

6. (C) The principal signs and symptoms of a dislocation are pain, loss of motion, and deformity. If a fracture were involved, swelling, ecchymosis, and grating or crepitus would be observed. With either a dislocation or a fracture, you always check pulses, muscle strength, and sensation distal to the injury. Treatment for either injury is also identical.

7. (A) Evaluation of distal pulses must be done in order to check the circulatory status of the involved extremity. Angulated fractures of joints are not straightened since to do so may cause further injury to the joint. A

sling and swathe would immobilize the fracture in the found position and prevent further injury. Although the application of a rigid splint will prevent a limb from bending or moving, it would require the angulation to be straightened. A padded board splint is a type of rigid splint.

8. (C) The posterior tibial pulse is found behind the medial malleolus. The popliteal artery (popliteal pulse) is located behind the knee where the joint flexes. The saphenous vein crosses in front of the medial malleolus. The dorsalis pedis pulse is found on the dorsum of the foot.

9. (C) Ligaments provide the majority of joint stability. They attach from bone to bone, are formed of collagen, and are very strong. Tendons move joints through a range of motion. Muscles provide skeletal motion. The joint capsule maintains the integrity of the joint but does not provide for joint stability.

10. (B) An open fracture refers to an opening or communication between the outside environment and the fracture site. Therefore an external object such as a bullet may cause an open fracture. Bone protruding through the skin is only one type of open or compound fracture. Open fractures may be reduced if circulation or neurological status is impaired, but not all such fractures are routinely reduced, and comminuted fractures exist when there are multiple bone fragments.

11. (D) Deformity may occur but is not nearly as common as pain, inability to move an extremity or joint, and swelling. Diagnosis of the type of injury must never be made on the absence of deformity.

12. (D) A fracture of the pelvis is most likely to produce the largest blood loss. Estimates of potential blood loss in the 6 hours after injury include the following: pelvis 1300–1500 cc; femur 400–800 cc; tibia-fibula 300–500 cc; humerus 150 cc.

13. (D) As intracranial pressure increases, arterial perfusion to the brain is decreased. In an attempt to force blood into this pressurized area, the systolic blood pressure rises and diastolic pressure decreases. There is then a reflex bradycardia. The paramedic should assess intracranial pressure changes by level of consciousness and pupillary changes rather than by vital signs, as changes in vital signs are a later development.

14. (C) Increasing intracranial pressure pushes a portion of the temporal lobe onto the brain stem, putting pressure on the reticular activating system and the oculomotor nerve located on the same side as the pressure. This pressure results in decreased level of consciousness and dilation of the pupil of the eye on the same side as the pressure on the oculomotor nerve.

15. (B) A patient in metabolic acidosis will exhibit Kussmaul breathing in an attempt to correct the acid-base imbalance. Cheyne-Stokes respirations may occur as a result of damage to the area just above the brain stem. Central neurogenic hyperventilation is often seen in the decerebrate patient and results from an injury to the pons and midbrain. Apnea may result from severe damage to or pressure on the brain stem.

16. (B) Extension of legs and flexion of arms (decorticate posturing) is assumed by patients with severe brain dysfunctions. A patient with spinal cord injury may assume any or none of the following positions: forearms flexed across chest, hands held above head, head tilted to one side.

17. (C) Until proven otherwise, all head injury patients should be managed as if they also have a spinal cord injury. Respiratory depression and blood loss may occur; however, these conditions are not present with all head injury patients.

18. (C) This situation describes the classic presentation seen with an epidural bleed, which usually includes an episode of unconsciousness followed by a lucid interval, followed by rapid deterioration. A subdural hematoma may progress more slowly following head injury, and may result in severe headache, nausea, nuchal rigidity, and finally coma. It can result from a blow to the temporal area, but the symptoms presented by the ball player are not those of a subdural hematoma.

19. (B) Rapid deterioration suggests an arterial bleed. The location of the injury is significant because the middle meningeal artery is located in the temporal area and, therefore, is vulnerable to trauma in this area.

20. (A) The signs of periorbital ecchymosis and bruising behind the ear, also called raccoon's eyes and Battle's sign, are classically associated with basilar skull fracture. Doll's eyes refer to a maneuver which is performed to determine the severity of the brain trauma. Watery drainage

refers to cerebral spinal fluid drainage which occurs when the arachnoid, dura, or the bone has been penetrated as a result of the injury.

21. (C) A subdural hematoma may occur as a very slow bleed with subtle neurological changes. If the patient is under the influence of alcohol, these signs/symptoms may be missed because of a decreased level of consciousness.

22. (C) The cervical and lumbar vertebrae do not have supportive protection and are most often injured. The thoracic vertebrae benefit from some splinting effect by the lungs.

23. (B) Bone fragments and disc displacement will cause pressure on the cord in varying degrees. Early intervention may prevent permanent damage. Depending on the mechanism, type of injury, and presence of other injuries, the patient may have little or no pain. Even without pain, the patient must be managed as if there is injury until proven otherwise. This patient requires special handling to prevent further injury.

24. (C) The patient with a spinal cord injury must be monitored closely for hypoventilation. The diaphragm is innervated by fibers of several cervical nerves which emanate from the phrenic nerve. When injury occurs at this level, breathing is affected.

25. (A) Loss of sympathetic tone (alpha receptor stimulation) will lead to widespread vasodilation and therefore significant heat loss. Conservation of heat must be part of the field management of the spinal cord-injured patient.

26. (C) Management includes oxygen, Narcan, dextrose, and spinal immobilization. Oxygen is provided for all patients at risk for hypoventilation. Narcan reverses the effects of a drug overdose, and dextrose increases the glucose level in hypoglycemic patients. These actions will produce a conscious state in patients with a drug overdose or insulin reaction. Spinal immobilization should also be provided for all patients for whom trauma cannot be ruled out. Benadryl is not appropriate as it is used for allergic reactions. Syrup of ipecac is never given to a patient with an altered LOC due to the risk of aspiration.

27. (B) Patients who hit their heads while diving into a pool frequently sustain high cervical cord injuries; therefore, this patient should be man-

aged as a spinal cord-injured patient until a complete assessment proves otherwise. The neurological examination should be completed after he has been stabilized. Intubation would not usually be the initial intervention. An IV is not the first priority with this patient.

28. (C) Immobilization must include both the cervical spine and the torso. If the body is not immobilized, it may slide or slip and put torque on the cervical area. Cervical immobilization takes special training and teamwork to perform. The use of traction with cervical immobilization is controversial in the field and the paramedic must know local standards regarding this action. C-collar application is *not* sufficient for true immobilization. The paramedic should report any movement of the patient before the arrival of the paramedic team but should still go ahead with spinal immobilization.

29. (D) Central neurogenic hyperventilation is caused by injury to the lower portions of the brain stem and is a late sign of brain herniation syndrome. Cheyne-Stokes respirations is a periodic increase and decrease in respiratory volume separated by periods of apnea. Kussmaul respirations, where breathing is increased in depth and rate, is the result of diabetic ketoacidosis. Eupneic ventilation is a normal respiratory pattern.

30. (A) While Battle's sign and blood flowing from the right ear indicate possible head injury, the patient's vital signs indicate a shock state. Since an isolated head injury will not cause shock, there must also be internal hemorrhage.

31. (B) Self-inflicted shotgun wounds typically bisect the face from the mandible through the forehead. The patient will have tremendous disfigurement and a severe airway problem that is best (or only) handled by the placement of the endotracheal tube. Good visualization of the vocal cords may be difficult, so watching for air bubbles can help you locate the tracheal opening. Once the tube is in place, pack 4 X 4s around the tube and all open wounds. Wrap the wound with elastic bandages to control bleeding.

32. (C) Application of direct pressure to the vessels above and below the point of a laceration will reduce the chance of an air embolism. A bulky dressing can be applied, but manual pressure on the vessels must be continued. Treat for shock as indicated. Transport the patient on the left

side with the head down about 15 degrees. Such a position will also reduce the dangers of an embolism. Dysrhythmia should be suspected, and the patient should be monitored. Do not apply circumferential bandages because they could interfere with circulation in the uninjured side of the neck.

33. (B) Situations such as the impalement of a knitting needle through the cheek are often dramatic but usually not serious unless airway obstruction is involved. Generally, an impaled object in the cheek should be removed in the same direction it entered. Once the object has been removed, the wound should be dressed on the inside as well as the outside in order to control bleeding. The patient should be positioned to allow any bleeding to drain from the mouth. Suction as required.

34. (B) Your first action in the treatment of open, soft tissue wounds should be to control bleeding. Prevention of further contamination and immobilization should follow the control of bleeding. Ice packs may be applied to closed wounds (contusions) to minimize edema and cause vasoconstriction. Elevation of an injured extremity above the level of the heart will also help control bleeding.

35. (C) Proper care for amputated body parts includes wrapping the part in a sterile dressing, placing it in a plastic bag, and placing the bag in an ice chest. The tissue should not be in direct contact with the ice. Avoid freezing the part (for example, with dry ice). Do not complete amputations even if the part is connected by only a few strands of tissue (skin bridge). Nerves and blood vessels may be intact, allowing better success if reimplantation is attempted. Bleeding from the stump can normally be controlled through the use of compression dressings. Avulsed teeth may be kept in a warm solution or in the patient's mouth if not contraindicated.

36. (B) Injuries to the abdomen where the viscera are protruding are managed by covering them with dressings soaked in saline solution. This treatment will prevent the organs from drying out and becoming necrotic. A moderately tight bandage is applied to keep the dressings in place.

37. (B) Trauma to the upper left quadrant with complaints of generalized abdominal pain would lead you to suspect that the spleen is involved.

As a general rule, abdominal disorders cannot be diagnosed or treated in the field. Your care for this patient would consist of treating the presenting signs and symptoms. Since the patient's signs and symptoms indicate he is in shock, shock is what you would treat. Oxygen by mask is preferred over the nasal cannula due to the ability of the mask to deliver a higher concentration of oxygen. The type of IV fluid administered will depend on the severity of the shock and local preference, but will usually be a crystalloid, like normal saline or lactated Ringer's, to run wide open. D_5W does not expand the blood volume. The IV is used as a keep-open line for giving medications to cardiac patients. In a supine position, the patient is lying on his back; with the legs slightly elevated, you are maintaining a physiological position. In a prone position, the patient would be lying face down and you would be unable to render care. The Trendelenburg's position causes further respiratory embarrassment and increases the work load of the heart. All patients in a shock state should be monitored for developing dysrhythmias. Vital signs are taken every 15 minutes and more frequently if needed to monitor the patient's shock state.

38. (B) As low-voltage electricity travels through the body from the contact point, it generates extreme heat that follows the path of the blood vessels and nerves. This heat can produce significant internal injury not obvious upon initial examination. High voltage has a tendency to take the shortest path rather than the one of least resistance. Alternating current (AC) produces more dangerous reactions than direct current (DC) since it can cause tetanic spasms (severe muscle contractions). Electrical burns often produce more extensive internal injury than burns to the integumentary system (skin).

39. (B) Kinetic energy is determined by the formula: one-half of the mass X velocity squared. Therefore the speed increases the production of kinetic energy more than the mass of the object. The type of automobile and restraints play a role in the absorption of energy and how much energy will be transferred to the patient, but do not affect the amount of energy in the collision.

40. (C) The ejected occupant has a six times greater chance of being killed than an occupant who stays with the vehicle. The occupant compartment absorbs the kinetic energy.

41. (D) The most important factor in "killing power" with penetrating trauma is the structure penetrated. The actual wound severity is a factor of kinetic energy and cavitation. Missiles of the greatest velocity cause a larger temporary cavity and damage beyond the path of the missile. Rifles usually have a greater muzzle velocity than handguns. The .44 Magnum has a velocity of 1470 ft/sec, and the M-14 has a velocity of 2610 ft/sec.

42. (A) Falls of greater than three times a person's height are usually severe. A fall that results in fractures of the ankles often causes compression injury to the spine. Liver and aortic injuries are usually associated with blunt deceleration injury to the anterior chest. The "hangman's" fracture usually results from direct axial loading of the cervical spine.

43. (A) Due to the obvious injuries and uncompensated shock this patient is a priority-1 trauma patient.

44. (B) Due to the catastrophic nature of the injuries, the chances of survival are slim. Placing the patient in a delayed category (P-2) will divert attention to more salvageable patients while ensuring him some level of care when it becomes available.

45. (A) Using most triage techniques, this child would be assessed last because he appears to be a priority 3, or walking wounded patient. However, the mechanism of injury and vital signs suggest hidden bleeding and compensated shock. This patient needs rapid intervention to survive. He should be treated as a priority 1.

46. (B) Since the patient is nonambulatory and has evidence of concussion and orthopaedic injury, she is a priority-2 patient.

47. (A) While tracheal deviation is a sign frequently discussed with tension pneumothorax, it is a late sign. Tachycardia, tachypnea, and diminishing breath sounds are earlier indicators.

48. (B) The angle of Louis is formed by the immovable joint of the manubrium and the sternal body and is useful in locating the second rib. Just lateral to either side are the second ribs. Once the second rib is located, the subsequent ribs and intercostal spaces are easier to identify. The

hypothenar eminence is in the palm of the hand. The point of maximal impulse is in the lower chest and marks the cardiac apex. The xiphoid process is at the inferior tip of the sternum.

49. (D) The dyspnea, pleuritic chest pain, mechanism of injury, and oximeter reading are suggestive of hypoxemia and pulmonary contusion. Hypoxia frequently causes cardiac dysrhythmias. Early correction of hypoxia is imperative. Cardiac contusion must also be suspected. There is no evidence of a pericardial tamponade and no history that supports the diagnosis of pulmonary embolism.

50. (D) Hypoxia can cause various cardiac dysrhythmias and is commonly associated with ventricular ectopy. Bundle branch block may be associated with injury to the conducting system in the ventricular septum. Injury to the myocardium can also result in ventricular ectopy.

51. (C) The vital signs do not indicate a need for volume challenge with crystalloid solution at this time. Additional volume may cause increased hypoxemia due to increased fluid leakage into the lung interstital space and impaired oxygen transfer in the lung.

52. (D) Monitoring the ECG is not an initial priority. Even though the wound appears to be in the abdomen, the path of the knife may have penetrated the pleura and caused a pneumothorax. Therefore, the wound should be sealed, and the patient should be provided with supplemental oxygen and volume replacement.

53. (B) Bleeding under the diaphragm may cause irritation and referred pain to the shoulder on the same side as the injury. Injuries to the spleen may cause referred pain to the left shoulder.

54. (B) Blood is not as irritating to the peritoneum as gastric juices, which typically cause involuntary guarding of the abdomen. Since you had no chance to assess the patient before injury and measure abdominal girth, it is difficult to use distension of the abdomen as a positive indicator of occult bleeding. Lack of guarding and/or distension does not rule out bleeding. Suspicion of abdominal trauma and bleeding must be based upon mechanism of injury, inspection of the abdomen, and palpation of the abdomen to elicit pain or discomfort.

55. (B) Auscultation of bowel sounds is not a useful prehospital diagnostic tool. To confirm presence or absence of sounds requires a minimum of several minutes of auscultation under quiet conditions. Inspection and palpation are standard techniques of physical assessment. Measurement of peripheral oxygen saturation is an immediate tool to determine how well the patient is oxygenated.

56. (B) The rib cage of a child is pliable and fractures are uncommon. Blunt trauma producing enough energy to fracture ribs has likely resulted in other injury. This patient must be treated as seriously injured.

57. (A) Unless contact lenses are removed, the sulfuric acid may find its way behind the lens and continue to burn and cause further damage to the eye. Flushing is done with copious amounts of water. Chemical antidotes are never used. Both eyes are bandaged in order to prevent sympathetic movement and further damage to the injured eye.

58. (B) Rose's burns cover approximately 36% of her body surface. Each arm is 9% (18% together), and half of each leg would be 9% (18% together). An adult head is 9%. The trunk is 18% front, 18% on the back.

59. (D) A severely burned patient should have all jewelry and other potentially constricting items removed as soon as possible since swelling of the fingers and hands may occur. Debris should not be picked from the skin. Adults will usually get an order for approximately 5–10 ml/kg body weight per hour of IV fluids. Neonates would typically have about 15 ml per hour infused, while infants 6 months to 1 year might receive 30 ml per hour of normal saline or Ringer's solution. High-concentration O_2 is indicated, especially if respiratory problems are suspected or present. Burns around the face, singed nasal hair, hoarseness, or cyanosis are all clues of potential respiratory burns. A patient burned in a closed space or unconscious in a burning area also has a strong risk of respiratory involvement. Intubation, even of the conscious, may be indicated if laryngeal edema develops. Rapid transportation is always indicated as burns can stop circulation if the area involved is circumferentially burned.

60. (B) Pain and redness involving the epidermis typify a first-degree burn. Blistered areas, or burns involving the dermis, are classified as second-degree burns. Charred areas, areas of pallor, or painless areas due to the death of the nerve endings, characterize third-degree burns.

61. (A) The bull's-eye type burn is typical of an extreme contact burn. Flash or arc burns usually cause extensive superficial injury. Flame burns from electricity are usually the result of clothing or other combustibles being set on fire by an arc or electrical current.

62. (C) Cameron has suffered extensive burns covering approximately 72% of his body. A child's head and neck are considered 18%. Each arm is 9% (18% together), and his entire torso is 36% (18% front and 18% back). Each leg is 13.5%.

63. (B) A second-degree burn involving 15 to 30% of the body surface is classified as a moderate burn; therefore this patient has the lowest priority for treatment. Most burns to the face, hands, feet, and genitalia are considered critical as loss of function could be devastating. Burns complicated by a fracture or a serious, pre-existing disease are also considered critical. Deep, second-degree burns should be considered critical as they are close to being third-degree burns.

64. (C) Dry lime is water-soluble and becomes corrosive when mixed with water. Therefore lime should be brushed away, not flushed with water. All jewelry and clothing should be removed in order to eliminate further burning from lime concealed under the jewelry or clothing. Once the dry chemical is brushed off, copious amounts of water can be used for irrigation. Sterile dressings should be applied to all burn areas in order to prevent contamination and subsequent infection.

65. (B) The head and neck combine for 9%. The chest is half of the anterior thorax (18%) which would also equal 9%. The anterior left leg would also equal 9% since the entire leg (posterior and anterior aspects) is 18%. Since each arm contributes 9%, both arms would equal 18%. This totals 45%.

66. (A) The Parkland Formula is used to determine the amount of fluid that the patient must be given during the first eight hours post-trauma and is as follows:

$$\frac{4 \text{ ml} \times \text{percent of body surface area burned} \times \text{patient's weight (kg)}}{2}$$

To convert pounds to kilos, divide pounds by 2.2 ($175 \div 2.2 = 80$).

Applying this formula to Mr. Banks is as follows:

$$\frac{4 \times 45 \times 80}{2} = \frac{14400}{2} = 7200 \text{ every 8 hours}$$

In order to deliver this volume, 900 ml must be given per hour. Dividing the gtts/ml (10) into 60 (minutes/hour) = 6. Six divided into 1080 (ml/hour) = 150 gtts/min.

67. (A) Assessment of the patient's potential injuries requires the paramedic to remember that electricity follows the path of least resistance throughout the body (e.g., nerves, blood vessels, etc.). The ability to trace the probable path of the current allows the paramedic to quickly identify and treat the patient's injuries. Because the extent of external injury is usually minimal compared to the internal damage, electrocution victims must be treated as critically injured patients. Alternating current (AC) is the most dangerous form of electricity because the intermittent surges of electrical energy cause tetanic spasms of the muscle which causes the individual to "freeze" to the source of energy. Direct current (DC) flows through the body without producing such muscle spasms.

68. (C) Due to the potential of hypothermia, wet dressings are used only on burns involving less than 10% BSA (Body Surface Area) or no more than 10% of BSA at a time. Since this patient has a gag reflex and is demonstrating signs consistent with hypoxia (restlessness being one of the first), blind nasotracheal intubation is recommended as the means of maintaining a patent airway and providing adequate oxygen therapy. Orotracheal intubation is not indicated due to the possibility of laryngospasm. Although morphine and nitrous oxide must be given cautiously to prevent hypotension and respiratory depression, analgesia would be appropriate therapy for this patient.

69. (C) Homeostasis is maintained at the capillary level through the relative balance of the pulling (from the vascular bed) and pushing (to the vascular bed) forces. These are as follows:
Blood to tissues (pulling force)
17.0 mm Hg—Capillary fluid pressure
 6.3 mm Hg—Interstitial fluid pressure
 5.0 mm Hg—Interstitial colloid pressure
28.3 mm Hg—Total pulling force

Tissue to blood (pushing force)
28.0 mm Hg—Plasma colloid pressure

The colloid osmotic pressure results from the inability of proteins to cross the semipermeable membrane and enter the interstitial space. In a normal state, there is always a slow trickle of water from the blood into the tissues due to the 0.3 mm Hg difference. Accumulation of this fluid in the interstitium does not occur, because it is returned to the blood-vascular system by the lymph system.

70. (B) Burns will result in the destruction of capillaries, which causes large open areas along the capillary wall rather than the semipermeable pores normally present. This allows a large influx of proteins and fluid from the intravascular compartment into the interstitium. Increased pressure on the lymph valves causes them to close and thereby prevents the return of plasma proteins to vascular circulation. Since the plasma colloid osmotic pressure is the only gradient that exerts an osmotic pull in the direction of the tissue to the blood, the loss of protein from the vascular bed causes the plasma colloid osmotic pressure to decrease resulting in rapid edema. This will also result in a rapid increase in the interstitial colloid pressure. The loss of protein and fluid from the vascular bed to the interstitium causes a decreased plasma colloid osmotic pressure which results in the development of shock.

71. (C) This patient is a prime candidate for upper airway burns since she was inhaling superheated air in an enclosed area. Whereas dry heat produces inhalation injuries which are almost always limited to the upper airway, gas or steam produces burns to the lower airway. When heat enters the airway, it disperses in the nasopharynx and upper airway, resulting in burn injuries and edema. If the patient has a gag reflex and spontaneous respirations, nasotracheal intubation should be accomplished as quickly as possible to prevent airway obstruction due to the progression of edema. Any patient whose history indicates exposure to heat and fumes in an enclosed space must be assumed to have airway burns, carbon monoxide poisoning, smoke inhalation injuries, or any combination thereof, until proven otherwise.

5 Medical Emergencies

Respiratory
Cardiovascular System
Endocrine System
Nervous System
Acute Abdomen
Anaphylaxis
Toxicology, Alcohol and Drug Abuse
Infectious Diseases
Environmental Injuries
Geriatrics/Gerontology
Pediatrics

Respiratory

1. The condition characterized by increased mucus production and a productive cough for more than three months out of the year for two consecutive years is called:

   A. Asthma.
   B. Emphysema.
   C. Status asthmaticus.
   D. Chronic bronchitis.

2. Which of the following conditions produce exercise intolerance and dyspnea in the patient with emphysema?

   A. Mucus plugs, atelectasis, and hypoxia.
   B. Bronchospasm and hyperinflated lungs.
   C. Inelasticity of lungs and decrease in alveolar surface area.
   D. Hypoxic drive resulting in chronic tachypnea.

3. Chronic Obstructive Pulmonary Disease (COPD) patients in acute respiratory failure primarily need:

   A. Oxygen to correct hypoxia.
   B. Epinephrine to relieve bronchospasm.
   C. Suctioning to remove mucus plugs.
   D. Albuterol to relieve bronchospasm.

4. For the COPD patient in a compensated state, which of the following is the usual precursor to acute respiratory failure?

   A. Spontaneous pneumothorax.
   B. Left heart failure.
   C. Pulmonary edema.
   D. Lower respiratory infection.

5. Which of the following conditions is most closely associated with hypoxic respiratory drive?

   A. Hyperventilation.
   B. Asthma.
   C. Chronic bronchitis.
   D. Carbon monoxide poisoning.

6. Patients with a long history of COPD are more prone to develop all of the following *except*:

   A. Left heart failure.
   B. Right heart failure.
   C. Barrel chest.
   D. Prominent accessory muscles.

7. While acquiring a history from an elderly female patient complaining of dyspnea, you ask if she has COPD. The patient denies any knowledge of it, but has not been to a doctor in 30 years. Which of the following would be most useful in detecting undiagnosed COPD?

   A. Skin color and nail beds.
   B. Barrel chest and a history of smoking.
   C. Rhonchi and expiratory wheezing.
   D. Evidence of left heart failure.

8. The daughter of the patient in the preceding question tells you that her mother has become increasingly irritable and has complained of frequent headaches over the past few weeks. The mother's ability to reason has become impaired, and the daughter has noticed other subtle personality changes. Which of the following is the most likely cause of these symptoms?

   A. Hypercarbia.
   B. Hypocarbia.
   C. Hypoxia.
   D. Hypertension.

9. Which of the following conditions is most apt to present with hypotension and hypoxia?

   A. Pulmonary embolism.
   B. Pulmonary edema.
   C. Acute asthma.
   D. Chronic bronchitis.

10. Which of the following best describes the pathophysiology of pulmonary embolism?

   A. Destruction of alveoli.
   B. Mucus plugs in the bronchioles.

C. Left ventricular failure.
D. A ventilation/perfusion mismatch.

11. A pulmonary embolism is most likely to develop from which of the following?

    A. Venous clot from an upper extremity.
    B. Clot in the arterial circulation.
    C. Venous clot from a lower extremity.
    D. Clot from a pulmonary vein.

12. The primary disorder in the acute asthmatic patient is:

    A. Destruction of alveoli.
    B. Hypoxic drive.
    C. Inelasticity of lungs.
    D. Bronchospasm.

13. An asthma attack that is not broken by repeated doses of epinephrine is called:

    A. Status asthmaticus.
    B. Severe asthma.
    C. Acute asthma.
    D. Terminal bronchospasm.

14. What is the primary focus of management of the acute asthmatic patient?

    A. ECG monitoring to detect S-T segment changes.
    B. IV therapy for administration of medications.
    C. Rehydration to clear mucus plugs.
    D. Relief of bronchospasm and improvement of ventilation.

15. Inhalation of which of the following is most likely to cause burns to the lower airway and lungs?

    A. Superheated air.
    B. Superheated steam.
    C. Phosgene gas.
    D. Carbon monoxide.

16. You are treating a 60-year-old female asthmatic in acute respiratory distress. Wheezing is auscultated apex to base anteriorly and posteriorly. She is able to talk without difficulty to give you her history. She has a previous history of stable angina for which she takes nitroglycerine prn. Appropriate field treatment for this patient would include which of the following?

    A. IV crystalloid and oxygen.
    B. IV crystalloid, oxygen, and 0.3–0.5 mg 1:1000 epinephrine SQ.
    C. IV crystalloid, oxygen, 0.7–1.0 mg 1:1000 epinephrine SQ, and 500 mg aminophylline IV drip.
    D. IV crystalloid, oxygen, and 3–5 mg 1:1000 epinephrine SQ.

17. When epinephrine is administered to an adult patient for relief of bronchospasm, the dosage is usually:

    A. 0.3 mg of 1:10,000 solution IV push.
    B. 0.3–0.5 mg of 1:1000 solution SQ.
    C. 0.7–1.0 mg of 1:1000 solution SQ.
    D. 3.0–5.0 mg of 1:1000 solution SQ.

18. Which of the following therapies reflects the current initial management of an acute asthma attack in the adult patient?

    A. Aminophylline 500 mg over 20 minutes, IV.
    B. Epinephrine 0.5 ml of 1:10,000 solution IV.
    C. Albuterol 0.5% solution, 0.5 ml nebulized.
    D. Methylprednisolone 125 mg IV.

19. When administering aminophylline for an acute asthmatic attack, the usual dose is:

    A. 100–200 mg over 40 minutes.
    B. 250–500 mg over 20 minutes.
    C. 250–500 mg over 60 minutes.
    D. 500–1000 mg over 20 minutes.

20. You have been called to see a 70-year-old male complaining of dyspnea for two days, with accompanying fever, chills, and productive cough. He has sharp chest pain with each cough and is in mild respiratory distress. He has a history of COPD. Physical exam reveals an elevated tem-

perature, rales, and rhonchi over the right lower lobe and dullness to percussion over that lobe. Vital signs are P 110, R 36, BP 160/90, ECG sinus tachycardia. Treatment for this patient would include which of the following?

A. Oxygen, IV crystalloid, Lasix 40–80 mg, and morphine.
B. Oxygen, IV crystalloid KVO, monitor, and transport.
C. Oxygen, IV crystalloid KVO, nitroglycerine, and lidocaine.
D. Oxygen, IV $D_50.45$ normal saline, epinephrine SQ, and amino-phylline.

21. You are transporting a patient who is in severe respiratory distress. In addition to monitoring respiratory status, a pulse oximeter is utilized. Pulse oximetry assesses which of the following?

A. PaO_2.
B. Oxygen saturation.
C. Hypercarbia.
D. Hypocarbia.

22. Which of the following terms is used to describe the condition of more than one rib fractured in more than one place, causing an unstable seg-ment?

A. Sucking chest wound.
B. Flail chest.
C. Pneumothorax.
D. Hemothorax.

23. You are treating an unconscious patient with chest trauma who is cyanotic and tachypneic. Examination reveals jugular venous disten-tion, right tracheal deviation, and no breath sounds in the left anterior chest. The left chest is hyper-resonant to percussion. Appropriate care for this patient would include which of the following?

A. Oxygen, intubation, and pericardiocentesis.
B. Oxygen, intubation, and left needle thoracostomy.
C. Oxygen, intubation, and right needle thoracostomy.
D. Oxygen, intubation, and hyperventilation by bag-valve device.

24. Which of the following statements best explains the reason atelectasis decreases arterial oxygen levels?

A. Cardiac output decreases.
B. Collapsed alveoli do not contain oxygen.

C. Respiratory dead space increases.
D. The patient's lungs become hyperinflated.

25. Pain resulting from rib fractures predisposes the patient to:

    A. Atelectasis.
    B. Bronchospasm.
    C. Bronchitis.
    D. Excessive mucus production.

26. You are treating an alert, but anxious, 20-year-old male who complains of dyspnea and a tingling sensation in his hands, feet, and face. The onset began while waiting in his dentist's office. Your examination reveals a pulse of 130, respiratory rate of 40, and hands and feet flexed from apparent muscle spasms. He has equal breath sounds bilaterally and no significant previous medical history. What is the most likely cause of the muscle spasm?

    A. Respiratory acidosis.
    B. Respiratory alkalosis.
    C. Petit mal seizure.
    D. Focal motor seizure.

27. The thoracic and abdominal cavities are separated by the:

    A. Intercostal muscles.
    B. Sternocleidomastoid muscles.
    C. Diaphragm.
    D. Rectus abdominus muscles.

28. The right lung is composed of:

    A. One lobe.
    B. Two lobes.
    C. Three lobes.
    D. Four lobes.

29. What is the normal PaO_2 and $PaCO_2$ in an adult who is breathing room air at sea level?

    A. PaO_2 120 torr, $PaCO_2$ 46 torr.
    B. PaO_2 90 torr, $PaCO_2$ 35 torr.
    C. PaO_2 46 torr, $PaCO_2$ 90 torr.
    D. PaO_2 200 torr, $PaCO_2$ 90 torr.

30. Which of the following conditions occur when arterial O_2 (PaO_2) falls below 50–60 torr (mm Hg)?

    A. Apnea.
    B. Dyspnea.
    C. Anoxia.
    D. Hypoxia.

31. Which of the following is usually the primary reason for an increase in the respiratory rate in a healthy individual?

    A. $PaCO_2$ decrease.
    B. $PaCO_2$ increase.
    C. PaO_2 decrease.
    D. PaO_2 increase.

32. The amount of physiologic "dead space" in the respiratory system of the average adult male is:

    A. 150 ml.
    B. 350 ml.
    C. 500 ml.
    D. 4500 ml.

33. The primary respiratory center is located in the:

    A. Medulla.
    B. Cerebral cortex.
    C. Cerebellum.
    D. Aortic arch.

34. The normal pH range for arterial blood is:

    A. 7.00–7.35.
    B. 7.00–7.80.
    C. 7.35–7.45.
    D. 7.45–7.80.

35. The peripheral chemoreceptors are most sensitive to changes in:

    A. Hydrogen ion concentration.
    B. $PaCO_2$.

C. PaO$_2$.

D. Osmolarity.

36. The average tidal volume in a normal adult at rest is:

    A. 250 ml.
    B. 500 ml.
    C. 750 ml.
    D. 1000 ml.

37. If a patient in respiratory distress has a respiratory rate of 20 and his tidal volume is 1100 ml, his minute volume would be:

    A. 1100 ml.
    B. 2000 ml.
    C. 11,000 ml.
    D. 22,000 ml.

38. Which of the following is the first step in the detailed assessment of the chest to determine respiratory status?

    A. Lung auscultation with the stethoscope.
    B. Percussion of the chest.
    C. Palpation of the chest.
    D. Inspection of the chest.

39. Which of the following respiratory patterns is depicted in the diagram below?

    A. Cheyne-Stokes breathing.
    B. Neurologic hyperventilation.
    C. Kussmaul's respiration.
    D. Eupnea.

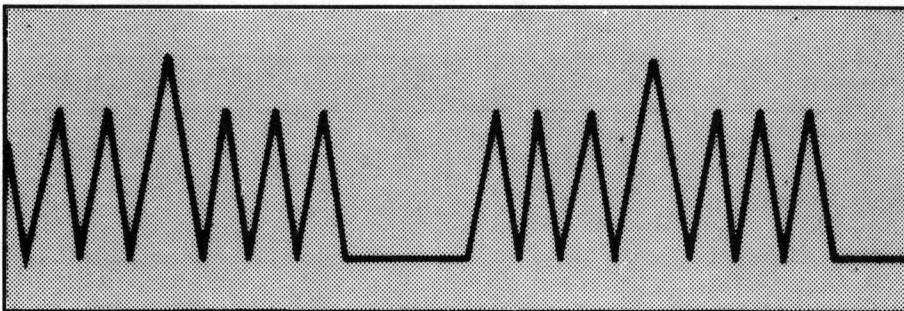

40. A patient with the respiratory pattern in the following diagram would have which of the following?

    A. Dyspnea.
    B. Eupnea.
    C. Biot's respirations.
    D. Kussmaul's respiration.

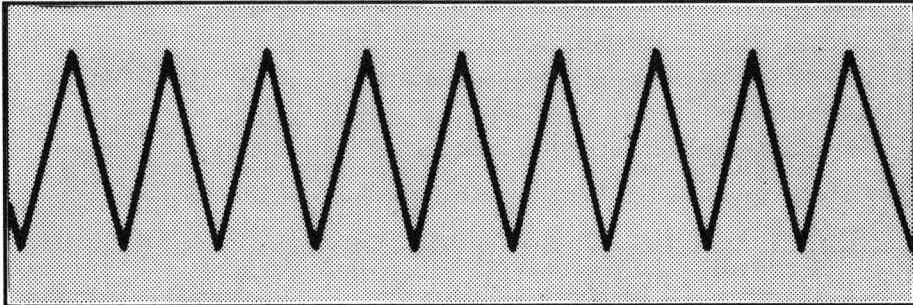

41. When auscultating the lungs, how should you instruct the patient to breathe?

    A. Normally, with the mouth open.
    B. Normally, with the mouth closed.
    C. Deeply, with the mouth open.
    D. Deeply, with the mouth closed.

42. Proper lung auscultation includes listening to breath sounds:

    A. For a full minute at each apex and base.
    B. For a full breath at apex and base posteriorly and anteriorly.
    C. At the posterior bases only.
    D. At the posterior apex only.

43. The type of breath sounds normally heard over most of the lung are:

    A. Bronchial.
    B. Broncho-vesicular.
    C. Vesicular.
    D. Tympanic.

44. Harsh, high-pitched sounds heard on inspiration and caused by upper airway obstruction are called:

    A. Rales.
    B. Wheezes.
    C. Stridor.
    D. Rhonchi.

45. Rales are best described as:

    A. Fine, moist sounds, heard on inspiration, that do not clear on coughing.
    B. Rumbling/rattling sounds on expiration that usually clear post-coughing or suctioning.
    C. Whistling/high-pitched sounds heard primarily on expiration.
    D. A loud or soft creak heard on inspiration and expiration.

46. A dyspneic patient complains of sharp chest pain in the upper right chest. It becomes worse on deep inspiration. Which condition is usually indicated by this type of pain?

    A. Acute bronchospasm.
    B. Pleuritic irritation.
    C. Acute myocardial infarction.
    D. Bronchial obstruction.

47. All of the following are objective physical signs of acute respiratory distress *except*:

    A. Frightened appearance.
    B. Flaring of nares.
    C. Intercostal muscle retraction.
    D. Feeling of shortness of breath.

48. In the normal, healthy adult, an arterial pCO_2 of 50 mm Hg would cause which of the following?

    A. Increased respiratory rate and depth.
    B. Decreased respiratory rate and depth.
    C. Increased respiratory rate and decreased depth.
    D. Decreased respiratory rate and increased depth.

49. Atelectasis occurs when the smallest unit of the respiratory system collapses, impairing gas exchange. Which anatomical structure is affected by atelectasis?

    A. Carina.
    B. Alveolus.
    C. Vallecula.
    D. Bronchiole.

50. Following head trauma, a patient may exhibit hyperpnea and tachypnea. This pattern of respiration is known as:

    A. Cheyne-Stokes respiration.
    B. Eupneic ventilation.
    C. Kussmaul's respiration.
    D. Central neurogenic hyperventilation.

51. Which of the following is *least* likely to be associated with a lower airway obstruction in the pediatric patient?

    A. Stridor.
    B. Wheezing.
    C. Nasal flaring.
    D. Intercostal retractions.

52. Which of the following figures correctly represents the percentage of oxygen in the atmosphere?

    A. 21%.
    B. 35%.
    C. 45%.
    D. 90%.

53. Your rescue unit responds to a man down in a restaurant. On arrival, the patient is unconscious and unresponsive. Foreign body aspiration is suspected. Following assessment and an unsuccessful attempt at ventilation, how many abdominal thrusts should be delivered in a series?

    A. 1–2.
    B. 3–4.
    C. 6–10.
    D. 20.

54. Your EMS unit is requested by a state patrol officer who has made a traffic stop for erratic driving. A 30-year-old male (the driver), his wife, and 4-year-old son are in the car. The officer reports that shortly after he

stopped the vehicle, the child suffered a grand mal seizure. The father denies that the child has been ill. The mother appears to be asleep. What is the most likely cause of the child's seizure?

A. Febrile seizure.
B. Idiopathic epilepsy.
C. Meningitis.
D. Carbon monoxide poisoning.

Cardiovascular System

55. Which valves are open during ventricular systole?

A. Mitral and aortic.
B. Mitral and tricuspid.
C. Aortic and tricuspid.
D. Aortic and pulmonic.

56. The smooth, epithelial, innermost layer of the heart is the:

A. Pericardium.
B. Endocardium.
C. Epicardium.
D. Myocardium.

57. The function of the chordae tendinae and papillary muscles is to:

A. Prevent backflow of blood into the ventricles.
B. Protect the coronary orifices when the aortic valve opens.
C. Prevent backflow of blood into the atrium.
D. Facilitate backflow of blood from the aorta.

58. Atherosclerosis is a disease process that affects the:

A. Tunica adventitia.
B. Tunica media.
C. Tunica intima.
D. Tunica externa.

59. The volume of blood ejected from the left ventricle into the arterial system each minute is:

A. Cardiac output.
B. Preload.
C. Stroke volume.
D. Afterload.

60. The period of time during the cardiac cycle when the myocardium will *not* respond to any stimulus is called the:

    A. Absolute refractory period.
    B. Frank-Starling mechanism.
    C. Relative refractory period.
    D. Electromechanical threshold.

61. Parasympathetic stimulation reduces the heart rate, the speed of impulses through the AV node, and the force of atrial contraction. This response is known as the:

    A. Adrenergic response.
    B. Cholinergic response.
    C. Anticholinergic response.
    D. Alpha-adrenergic response.

62. Normal impulse conduction through specialized tissues in the heart begins with the SA node and progresses in what order?

    A. AV node; internodal pathways; AV bundle; bundle branches; Purkinje system.
    B. AV bundle; internodal pathways; bundle branches; AV node; Purkinje system.
    C. Purkinje system; AV node; internodal pathways; bundle branches; AV bundle.
    D. Internodal pathways; AV node; AV bundle; bundle branches; Purkinje system.

63. When the tricuspid valve is closed, backflow of blood cannot enter the:

    A. Right atrium.
    B. Right ventricle.
    C. Left atrium.
    D. Left ventricle.

64. ECG markings relate to specific electrical events within the heart. Select the statement which correctly identifies these relationships.

    A. P-wave: atrial depolarization; QRS: ventricular depolarization; ST-T: ventricular repolarization.
    B. P-wave: atrial repolarization; QRS: ventricular depolarization; ST-T: ventricular repolarization.

C. P-wave: atrial depolarization; QRS: ventricular repolarization; ST-T: ventricular depolarization.

D. P-wave: atrial repolarization; QRS: ventricular depolarization; ST-T: ventricular depolarization.

65. Which term describes the gradual formation of a secondary or accessory blood supply for circulation to the heart?

A. Coronary.
B. Extracorporeal.
C. Collateral.
D. Lymphatic.

66. Which blood vessel supplies circulation to the majority of the left ventricular myocardium, a portion of the right ventricle, and the interventricular septum?

A. Posterior descending coronary artery.
B. Circumflex coronary artery.
C. Left main coronary artery.
D. Right main coronary artery.

67. The ability of certain cardiac cells to initiate excitation impulses spontaneously is called:

A. Automaticity.
B. Contractility.
C. Conductivity.
D. Excitability.

68. Which of the following statements concerning norepinephrine (Levophed) is *not* true?

A. Norepinephrine infiltration can cause tissue necrosis and sloughing.
B. Norepinephrine is a potent Alpha sympatholytic.
C. Norepinephrine is contraindicated in the presence of hypovolemic shock.
D. Norepinephrine administration is accomplished by a continuous IV infusion.

69. You are assigned to cover a weekend track and field event. One of the trainers is concerned about a 25-year-old marathon runner and asks you to check him out. His respirations are 18 per minute; his blood pressure is 130/80. The ECG reveals the following pattern:

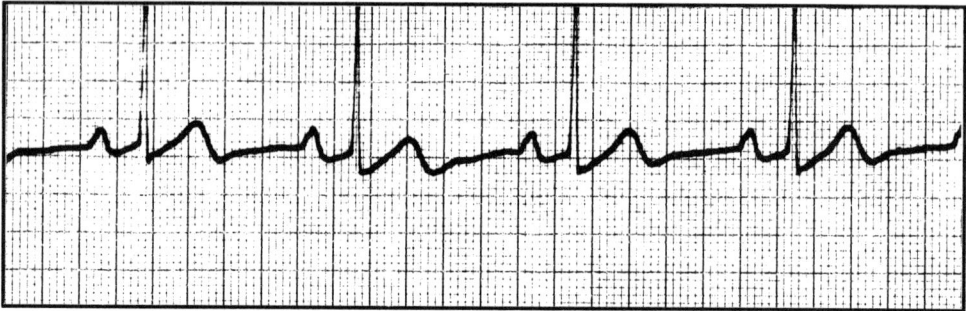

What is the appropriate action?

A. Administer atropine sulfate 0.5 mg IV.
B. Do nothing as this is a normal ECG for him.
C. Instruct the trainer to have the runner see his physician.
D. Administer oxygen at 6 L/min.

70. You are managing a patient in cardiac arrest. An endotracheal tube has been inserted. You are having difficulty establishing an IV line. You wish to administer epinephrine. What is the most appropriate action?

A. Administer 0.5 mg, 1:10,000 solution, subcutaneously.
B. Administer 1.0 mg, 1:1000 solution, subcutaneously.
C. Instill 0.5 mg, 1:1000 solution directly into the endotracheal tube.
D. Instill 1.0 mg, 1:10,000 solution directly into the endotracheal tube.

71. You respond to a call from a nursing home where the nurse tells you an elderly patient fainted but seems all right now. You obtain the following ECG:

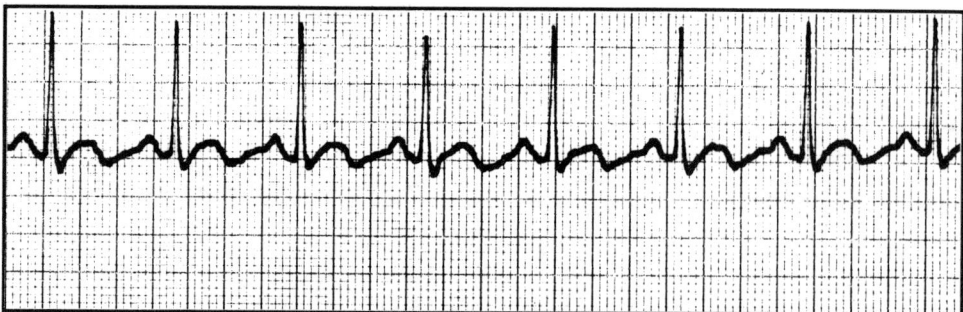

What is your interpretation?

A. First-degree AV block.
B. Second-degree AV block (Wenckebach).
C. Sinus arrhythmia.
D. Normal sinus rhythm.

72. A 58-year-old female was found unresponsive, apneic, and pulseless by a neighbor approximately 4 minutes prior to your arrival. Advanced cardiac life support was initiated and has been in progress for approximately 15 minutes with no response to therapy. The patient's ECG has remained unchanged throughout and is as follows:

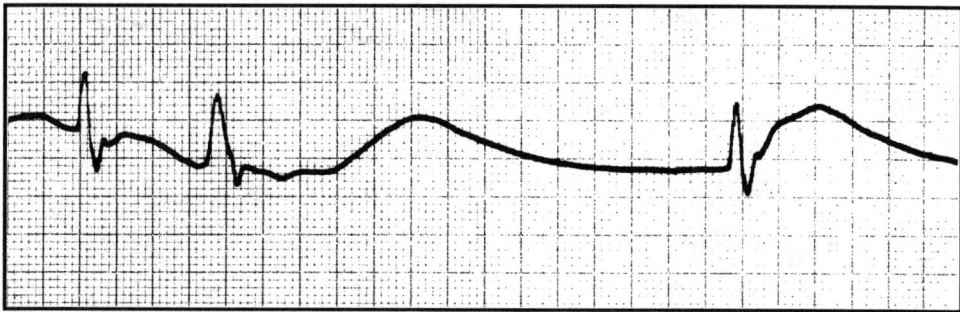

The next step in the management of this patient would be to administer:

A. A 200–500 ml fluid challenge of normal saline.
B. A bolus of 100 mEq of sodium bicarbonate IV.
C. Endotracheal epinephrine if there is no response to IV epinephrine.
D. Atropine sulfate 1.0 mg rapid IV push.

73. Which one of the following statements is *not* true about the cardiac cycle?

A. The electrical process of depolarization results in myocardial contraction.
B. The sinoatrial node (SA) discharges at a rate of 40–50 times per minute.
C. The cardiac cycle normally repeats every 0.8 seconds.
D. Ventricular filling decreases as the heart rate increases.

74. Mr. Evans is a 56-year-old construction supervisor. The company nurse called EMS when he began to complain of nonspecific, substernal heaviness while assisting his crew. He has no significant past medical history and takes no medications on a regular basis. Examination reveals a 170-pound male in obvious distress. His skin is pale and slightly diaphoretic. Although Mr. Evans appears apprehensive, he denies any shortness of breath. His BP is 100/70 and respirations are 28. His ECG is as follows:

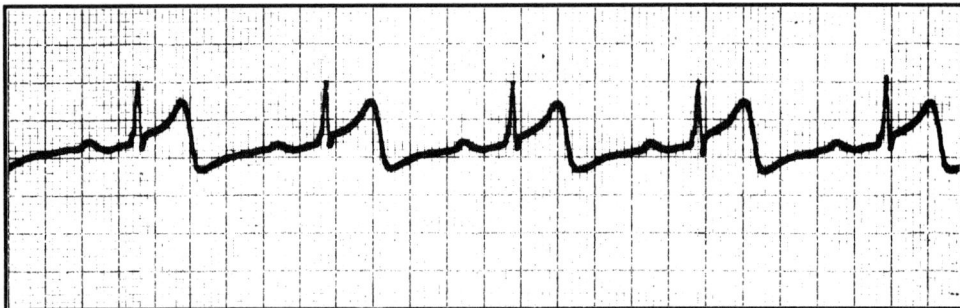

You suspect Mr. Evans is suffering from which of the following?

A. Heat exhaustion.
B. Dissecting aortic aneurysm.
C. Unstable angina pectoris.
D. Acute myocardial infarction.

75. Which of the following would *not* be indicated in the prehospital management of Mr. Evans?

A. Nitroglycerin 0.4 mg, repeated at 5 minute intervals X 3.
B. Oxygen administration at 6 liters per minute via nasal cannula.
C. Lidocaine 1.5 mg/kg IV followed by an infusion of 2 mg/min.
D. Continuous monitoring of the electrocardiogram.

76. Which of the following statements about defibrillation is not true?

A. Transthoracic resistance decreases with repeated countershocks.
B. The variable body sizes of adults must be considered when selecting the energy level.
C. Initially, three shocks should be administered if no change in rhythm occurs.
D. The availability of rapid defibrillation is the major determinant of survival in cardiac arrest secondary to ventricular fibrillation.

77. What is the correct position of the paddles for defibrillation?

     (1) Lateral the right nipple.
     (2) Lateral the left nipple.
     (3) To the right of the upper sternum and below the clavicle.
     (4) To the left of the upper sternum and below the clavicle.
     (5) Over the myocardial base at the 5th intercostal space.

     A. 1, 4.
     B. 2, 3.
     C. 2, 4.
     D. 2, 5.

78. A 74-year-old female called the ALS service because she is experiencing severe dyspnea. Physical examination reveals JVD, 4+ peripheral edema, and bibasilar rales. Respirations are 38 and labored; BP is 150/80. The ECG tracing obtained from the patient is as follows:

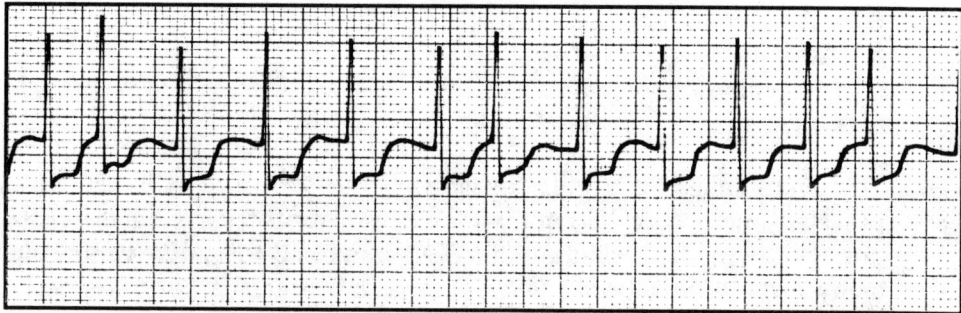

You interpret this rhythm as:

A. Sinus tachycardia with PACs.
B. Atrial flutter.
C. Second-degree AV block Type I.
D. Atrial fibrillation.

79. Which medication is most appropriate for the patient in the preceding question?

A. Morphine sulfate.
B. Diazepam.
C. Verapamil.
D. Propranolol.

80. You are called to see a 43-year-old male who is complaining of crushing, midsternal chest pain that began approximately 20 minutes ago. He is alert, pale, warm, and diaphoretic. The pain is so intense that he is extremely restless and apprehensive. Respirations are 26 and shallow; blood pressure is 110/80. His ECG is as follows:

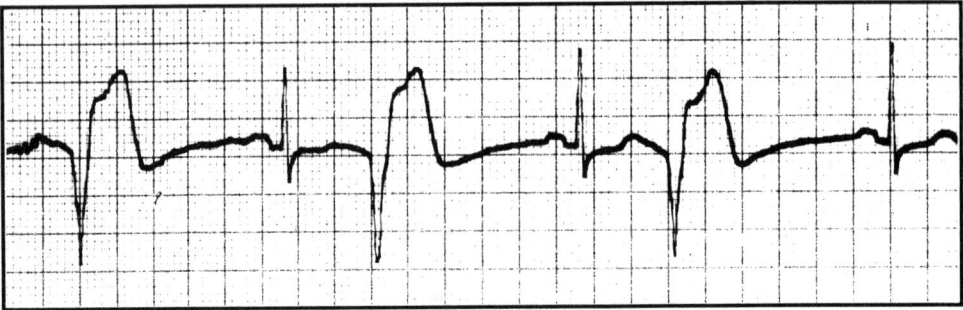

What is the first drug that should be administered to this patient?

A. Lidocaine.
B. Atropine.
C. Morphine sulfate.
D. Oxygen.

81. You were called to a golf course for a 63-year-old male who was pulseless and apneic. The quick-look demonstrated ventricular fibrillation. Following defibrillation, his ECG converted to a supraventricular tachycardia with a strong pulse. You administered a lidocaine bolus, followed by a lidocaine drip at the appropriate dose per minute. Prior to transport, you note the following ECG:

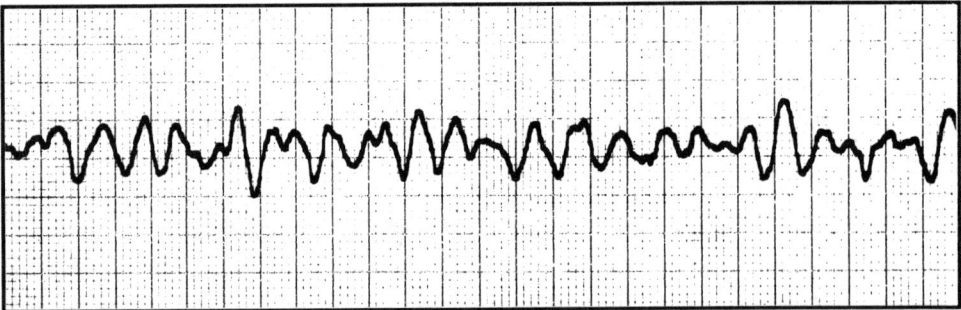

The pharmacological agent of choice at this time is:

A. Bretylium tosylate 5 mg/kg IV push.
B. Procainamide hydrochloride 20 mg/min IV slowly.

    C. Propranolol hydrochloride 1–3 mg every 5 minutes.
    D. Lidocaine hydrochloride drip increased to 4 mg/min.

82. Which of the following statements regarding sodium bicarbonate therapy is *not* true?

    A. Sodium bicarbonate does not improve the ability to defibrillate ventricular fibrillation.
    B. Sodium bicarbonate shifts the oxyhemoglobin saturation curve, inhibiting the release of oxygen.
    C. When sodium bicarbonate is indicated, half the initial dose is given every 5 minutes at the discretion of the team leader.
    D. Sodium bicarbonate produces paradoxical acidosis due to production of carbon dioxide, which is freely diffusible into myocardial and cerebral cells and may depress function.

83. Mr. Coyle is 47 years old and weighs 165 pounds. He began to experience midsternal chest pain after jogging last night. This morning the pain became more severe and was associated with nausea and diaphoresis. Respirations are 24/shallow; BP is 78/40. Pulse rate corresponds to the following ECG:

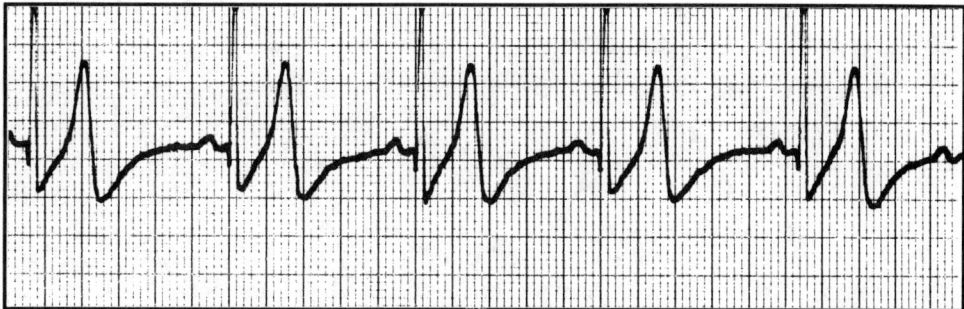

What is the initial pharmacological intervention required in this situation?

    A. Lidocaine 112.5 mg IV followed by a maintenance drip of 3 mg/min.
    B. Dobutamine (1000 mg mixed into 250 ml D_5W) at 28 microdrops per minute.
    C. Dopamine (800 mg mixed into 500 ml D_5W) at 14 microdrops per minute.
    D. Norepinephrine (1 mg mixed into 250 ml D_5W) at 30 microdrops per minute.

84. Mr. Welch (60 years old) called your ALS service because he has been experiencing nonradiating chest pain for approximately 2 hours. He describes the pain as a tight, oppressive sensation. The patient is restless and apprehensive. He is alert, pale, warm, and slightly diaphoretic. His pulse is 86/strong, respirations 20/min, BP 160/90. He denies any other associated discomfort and has no pertinent past medical history. The analgesic of choice in this situation is:

   A. Tridil 10 mcg/min titrated IV.
   B. Nitroglycerin 0.4 mg sublingually.
   C. Morphine sulfate 2–5 mg titrated IV.
   D. Amrinone 0.75 mg/kg titrated IV.

85. Mrs. Carey is complaining of shortness of breath, sudden weight gain, palpitations, and ankle edema. Medical Control has ordered you to administer IV furosemide. Mrs. Carey, who weighs 121 pounds, would require what initial IV dose of furosemide?

   A. 2.5–5.0 mg.
   B. 27.5–55 mg.
   C. 40–80 mg.
   D. 50–1000 mg.

86. How much pressure should be applied to defibrillator paddles when defibrillation is attempted?

   A. 10 pounds.
   B. 15 pounds.
   C. 20 pounds.
   D. 25 pounds.

87. You are called to the scene of a "man down." You apply the quick-look paddles and identify ventricular fibrillation. After defibrillation, you note the following rhythm:

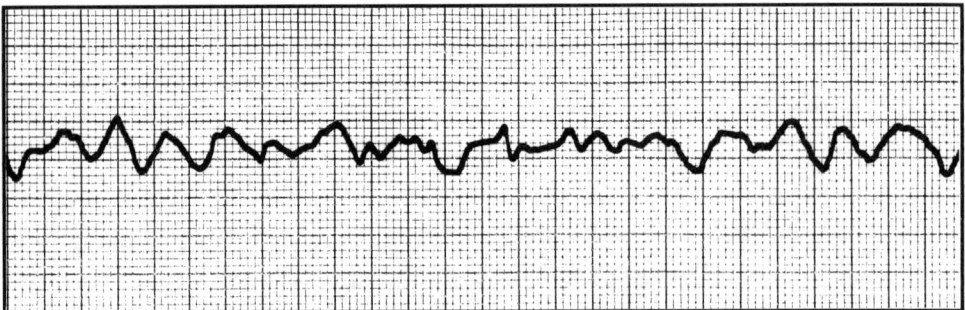

What is the next appropriate action?

A. Repeat the defibrillation.
B. Administer a lidocaine bolus IV push.
C. Ascertain if a carotid pulse is present.
D. Attach the ECG leads for further evaluation.

88. Calcium chloride is potentially indicated in all of the following situations *except*:

A. Hyperkalemia.
B. Hypocalcemia.
C. Verapamil toxicity.
D. Digitalis toxicity.

89. Which statement is *incorrect* regarding application of monitoring electrodes?

A. For continuous monitoring, ECG leads I, II, or MCL_1 may be used.
B. The ground electrode must be placed over the apex of the heart or under the right clavicular area.
C. For Lead II, the negative electrode is placed on the right upper chest.
D. For Lead MCL_1 , the negative electrode is placed on the left upper chest.

90. You are administering care to a patient who has the following ECG:

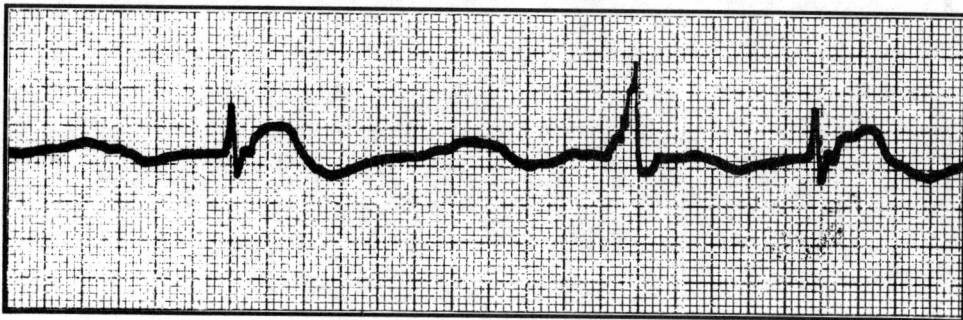

What is the most appropriate initial pharmacologic intervention?

A. Lidocaine 1 mg/kg IV push.
B. Atropine 0.5 mg IV push.
C. Isuprel 2–10 mcg/min IV piggyback.
D. Intropin 2–10 mcg/kg/min IV piggyback.

91. You are transporting a 28-year-old female who began to experience chest pain after consuming cocaine at a party. Her ECG is as follows:

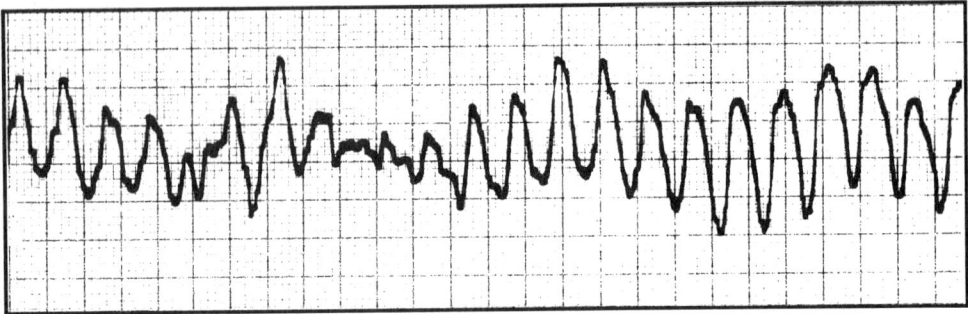

This dysrhythmia is identified as:

A. Torsade de pointes.
B. Ventricular tachycardia.
C. SVT with ventricular aberrancy.
D. Ventricular fibrillation.

92. A 72-year-old male called because he "just wasn't feeling well." He states he has had the flu for the past three days. His ECG is as follows:

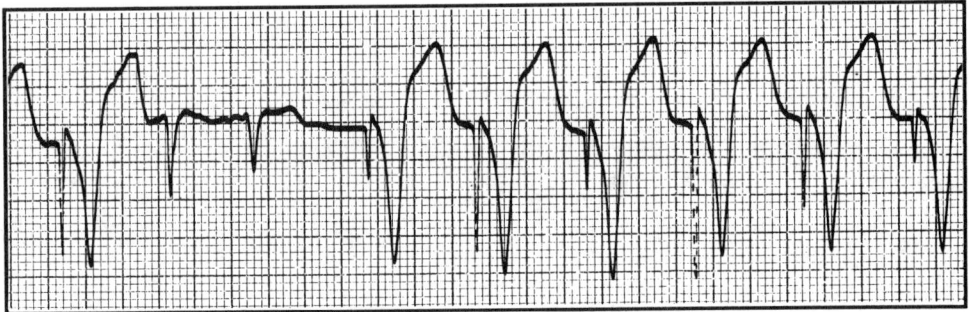

Which of the following is the most appropriate intervention for this dysrhythmia?

A. None.
B. Isuprel.
C. Lidocaine.
D. Bretylium.

93. A 56-year-old male called EMS because his "heart was racing." Although he is alert and oriented, his skin is pale, cool, and dry. He denies chest pain, dyspnea, or nausea. The past medical history includes an aortic valve replacement approximately 3 weeks ago. You are unable to palpate a BP. His carotid pulse is weak and palpable at 120/min. The ECG shows the following:

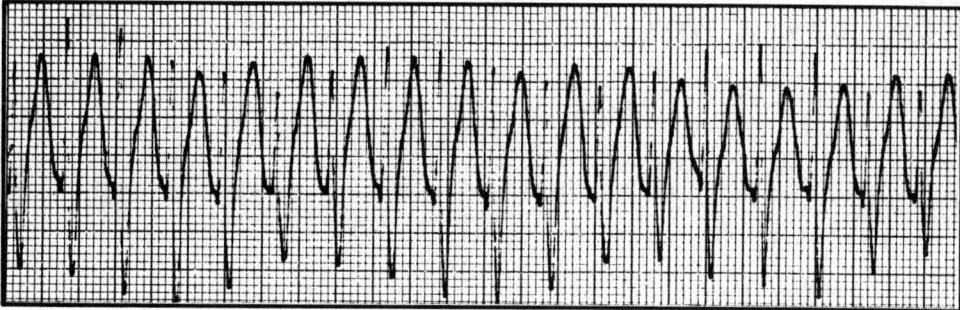

What is the initial management of this patient?

A. Synchronized cardioversion at 75–100 joules.
B. Vagal maneuvers such as the Valsalva maneuver.
C. Intravenous administration of Verapamil 5 mg.
D. Administration of a Beta blocker such as propranolol.

94. Your patient is a 65-year-old male complaining of substernal pressure. He is conscious and alert; pupils are PERL; skin is warm and slightly diaphoretic. Respirations are regular at 24/min, blood pressure is 110/60. He denies history of heart disease or similar episodes of this nature. His initial ECG is as follows:

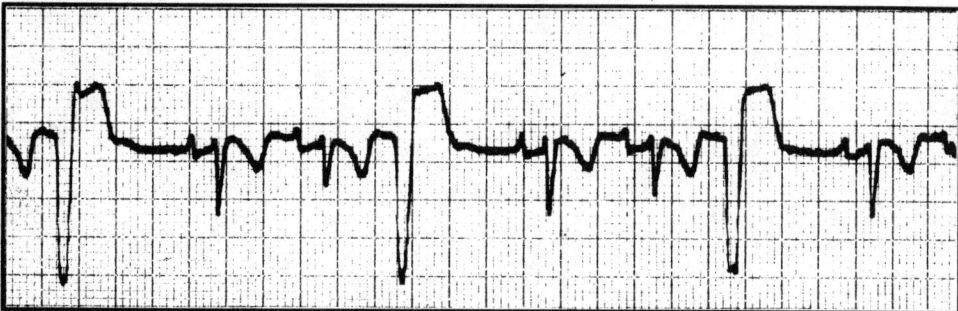

Utilizing your protocols, you administer the maximum dose of the drug of choice for this dysrhythmia. You now observe the following rhythm:

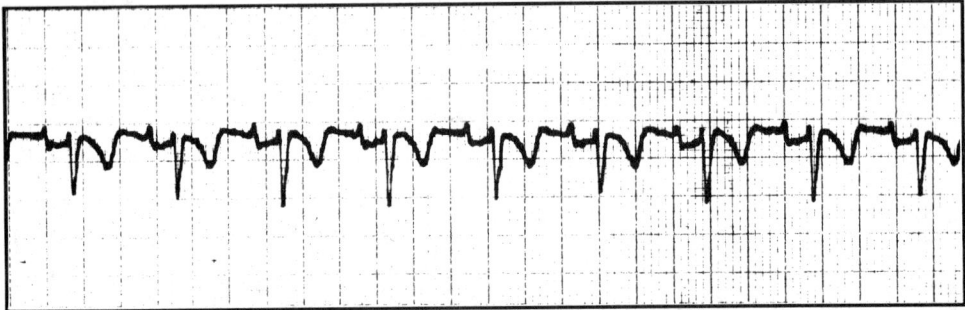

What is the next step in continuing care for this patient?

A. Lidocaine 4 mg/min IV piggyback.
B. Atropine 0.5 mg IV push.
C. Procainamide 1–4 mg/min IV piggyback.
D. Bretylium 2 mg/min IV piggyback.

95. Identify the following dysrhythmia:

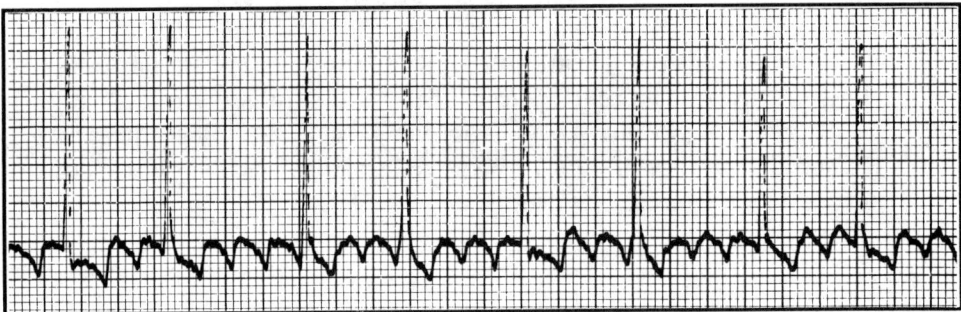

A. Supraventricular tachycardia.
B. Atrial fibrillation.
C. Atrial flutter.
D. Atrial tachycardia with block.

96. Which of the following medications possess both Alpha and Beta agonist properties?

     A. Isoproterenol, propranolol, and norepinephrine.
     B. Dobutamine, isoproterenol, and epinephrine.
     C. Epinephrine, digitalis, and sodium nitroprusside.
     D. Dopamine, norepinephrine, and epinephrine.

97. The Medical Control physician has ordered you to administer Nitronox to a patient for relief of atraumatic chest pain. You know that the maximum dose of Nitronox has been administered when the patient:

     A. Drops the hand-held mask.
     B. Receives 15 L/min for 2–3 minutes.
     C. Reports a euphoric sensation.
     D. Complains of nausea and dizziness.

98. Mrs. Marcum (36 years old) is complaining of "fluttering in her chest." Although she denies chest pain, she appears to be quite apprehensive. Her skin is pale, cool, and dry. Vital signs are pulse 120 and weak, respirations 30 and nonlabored, and BP 104/60. Her ECG is as follows:

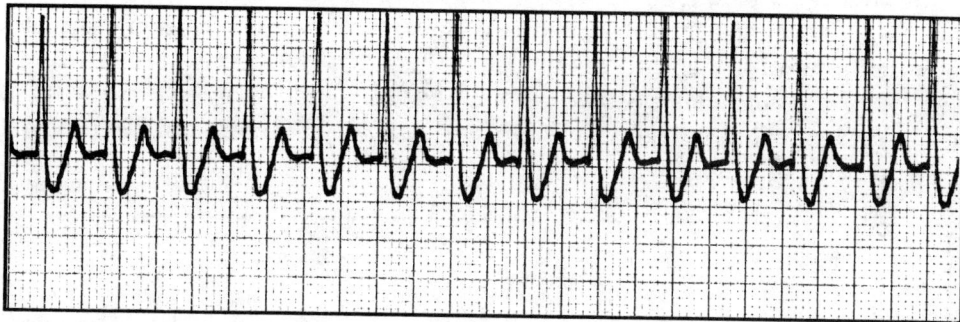

The discrepancy between the pulse and the ECG is due to which of the following?

     A. Decreased cardiac preload.
     B. Physiological AV dissociation.
     C. Increased diastolic time.
     D. Inadequate cardiac filling.

99. While rendering care to a patient who receives hemodialysis on an outpatient basis, you note the following ECG:

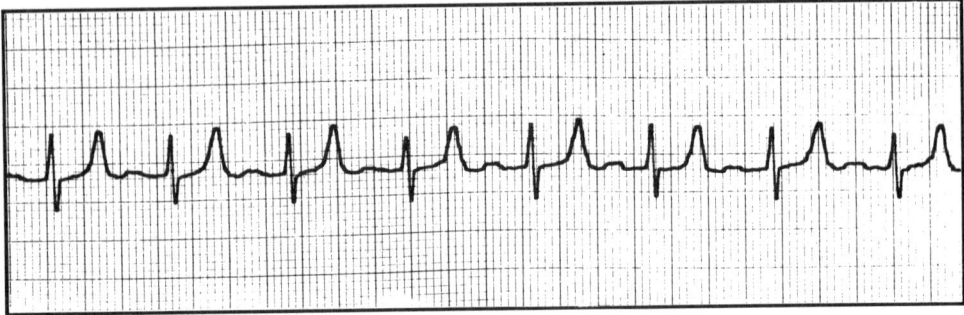

The predominant abnormality in this ECG is most likely due to:

A. Hypokalemia.
B. Hyponatremia.
C. Hyperkalemia.
D. Hypernatremia.

100. Joan, a 39-year-old female, called EMS because she experienced a sudden onset of chest pain. She is pale, cool, and clammy. JVD is noted at 45°. The patient reports that the pain is nonradiating and aggravated by respirations. She informs you that she had a hysterectomy two weeks ago and has not felt well since then. As you initiate oxygen therapy, Joan becomes unresponsive, apneic, and pulseless. Quick-look reveals the following ECG:

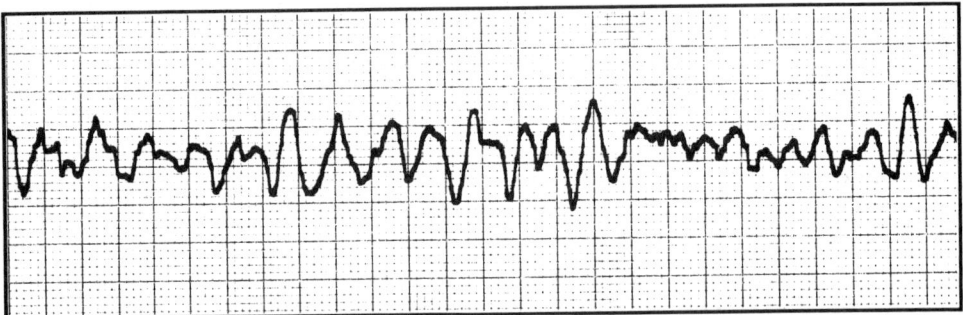

You suspect that this patient has experienced which of the following?

A. Pulmonary embolism.
B. Acute myocardial infarction.
C. Dissecting aortic aneurysm.
D. Spontaneous pneumothorax.

101. Your patient is a 68-year-old male whose chief complaint is generalized weakness. His medications include Lanoxin, Slo-K, and Lasix. He states that he does not take the Lasix on a regular basis because he has been golfing frequently and does not like the inconvenience caused by the medication. His ECG is as follows:

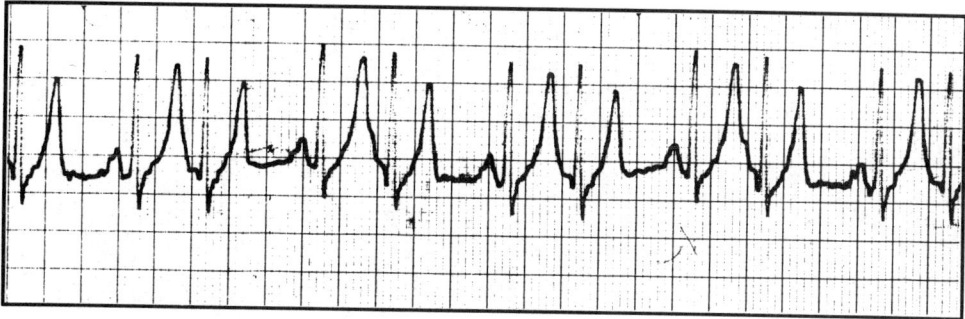

You would identify this dysrhythmia as:

A. Atrial bigeminy.
B. Sinus arrhythmia.
C. Atrial fibrillation.
D. Wandering atrial pacemaker.

102. Mrs. Tates (43 years old) is being transported to the hospital by your ALS unit. She is being admitted for chronic cardiomyopathy. Her ECG is as follows:

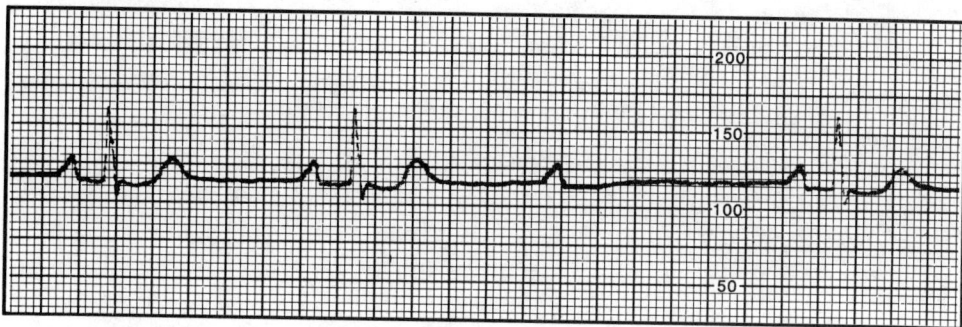

What is the correct interpretation of this dysrhythmia?

A. Third-degree heart block.
B. Second-degree AV block Type II.
C. Second-degree AV block Type I.
D. Sinus bradycardia with first-degree heart block.

Questions 103–106 relate to the following situation:

You are called to see a 100-kg, 47-year-old male who complains of retrosternal pressure, of sudden onset, for 20 minutes duration. His discomfort is not modified by movement, position, respiration, or palpation of the chest. There was no provocation to the event. He has a previous history of angioplasty 18 months ago and was prescribed nitroglycerin to take if needed. He has taken 4 prior to the arrival of EMS and complains of a headache presently. His pulse is 90, respirations 30, BP 98/palpation, SpO₂ 98. The ECG is as follows. His chest is clear bilaterally and there is no evidence of left or right heart failure. He is very apprehensive, restless, extremely pale, and diaphoretic.

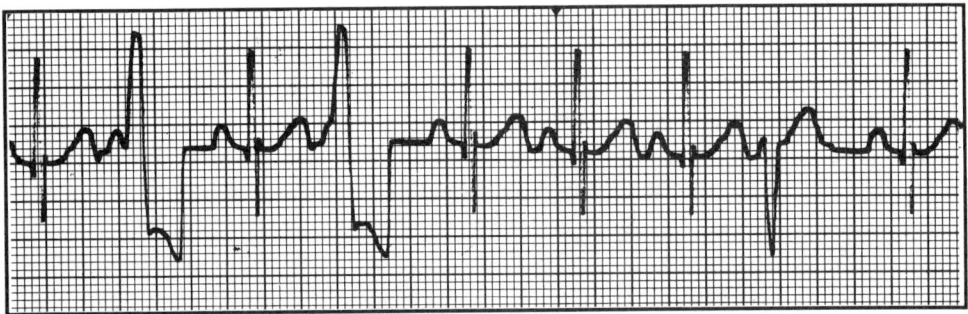

103. Your ECG interpretation is:

    A. Sinus rhythm with PVCs.
    B. Atrial fibrillation.
    C. Wandering atrial pacemaker.
    D. Sinus rhythm with PACs.

104. Your initial efforts to control pain should include:

    A. Nitroglycerin 0.4 mg sublingual.
    B. Morphine sulfate IV in 2-mg increments.
    C. Oxygen at 6 L/min by nasal cannula.
    D. Oxygen at 10 L/min by nonrebreathing mask.

105. What is the most appropriate initial approach to this situation?

    A. Establish an IV and a dopamine drip at 1–2 mcg/kg/min.
    B. Establish an IV, bolus with lidocaine 100 mg, and start a lidocaine drip at 4 mg/min.

C. Establish an IV, place the patient supine, and continue to monitor.
D. Establish an IV and a dopamine drip at 2–10 mcg/kg/min.

106. Which of the following statements most correctly describes this clinical situation?

   A. Stable angina and hypotension due to the nitroglycerin.
   B. Unstable angina and hypotension due to cardiogenic shock.
   C. Ischemia and hypotension due to the accelerated cardiac rate.
   D. Myocardial infarction and hypotension due to the nitroglycerin.

Questions 107–109 relate to the following situation:

You are called to a bus station to see a 55-year-old male who fainted while exiting a bus. He is responsive now and complains of chest pain. It is very difficult to communicate with him because he speaks broken English. The chest pain appears to have preceded the episode of syncope which occurred when he stood to exit the bus. He describes the pain as being in the center of his chest and radiating to his back. There is no evidence of a seizure. He has a history of hypertension and takes an unknown medication. He is pale, diaphoretic, and apprehensive. Vital signs are radial pulse 110–120 (easily palpated in the left arm, difficult to palpate in the right arm); respirations 30; BP 130/92; SpO$_2$ 94. The ECG is as follows. Lungs are clear and there is no JVD or dependent edema.

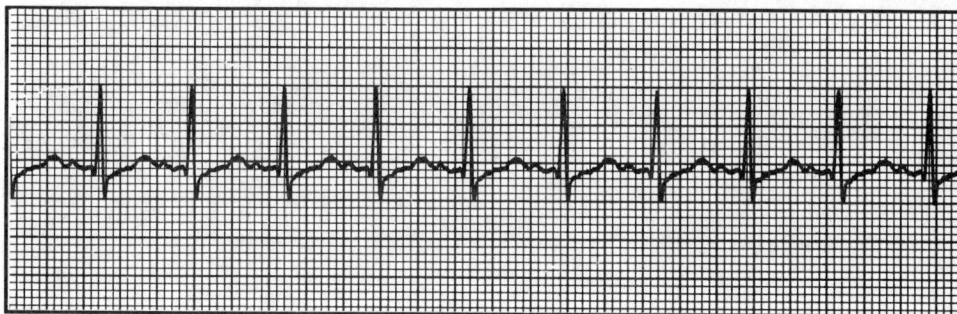

107. ECG interpretation is:

   A. Supraventricular tachycardia.
   B. Sinus tachycardia.
   C. Paroxysmal supraventricular tachycardia.
   D. Sinus rhythm.

The patient is moved to the ambulance because of the crowd and situation. You have started him on oxygen and established IV access. Vitals are reassessed: radial pulse is not palpable, respirations 36, BP 90/palpation, SpO₂ is unobtainable. ECG is as follows:

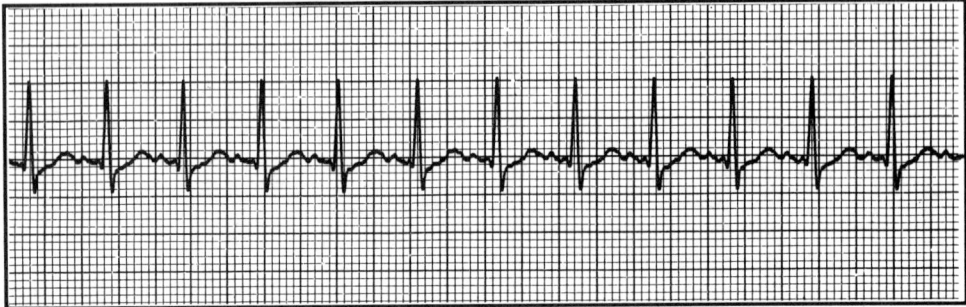

108. What is the most appropriate initial intervention?

    A. Vagal maneuvers to terminate the tachycardia.
    B. Verapamil 5 mg IV bolus.
    C. Synchronized cardioversion, after sedation.
    D. Fluid challenge with crystalloid solution and consider PASG.

109. Which of the following statements most correctly describes this clinical situation?

    A. Supraventricular tachycardia caused a Stokes-Adams attack.
    B. Supraventricular tachycardia is causing poor cardiac output and ischemia.
    C. Sinus tachycardia is causing poor cardiac output and ischemia.
    D. Sinus tachycardia is secondary to hypovolemia.

Questions 110–113 relate to the following situation:

You are called to see a 70-year-old female who complains of shortness of breath on exertion and a "funny" feeling in her chest. She has been previously healthy except for hypertension. When questioned about her discomfort, she describes it as a fullness or pressure in her chest. Vital signs are respirations 24, BP 166/88, SpO₂ 92. The ECG is as follows. Lungs are clear and there is no JVD or dependent edema.

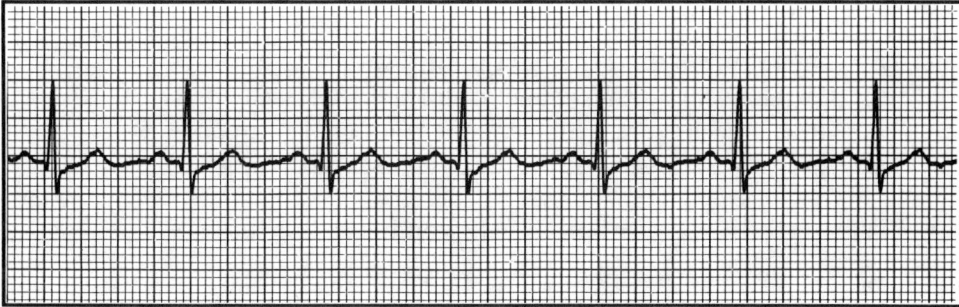

110. Your initial management for this patient would include which of the following?

    (1) Oxygen by nasal cannula.
    (2) Oxygen by nonrebreathing mask.
    (3) IV with lactated Ringer's.
    (4) IV with D_5W.

    A. 1, 4.
    B. 2, 4.
    C. 1, 3.
    D. 2, 3.

111. What is the most appropriate drug for the initial management of ischemic chest pain?

    A. Nitroglycerin 0.4 mg.
    B. Morphine 2 mg IV in increments.
    C. Morphine 5 mg IM.
    D. High-concentration oxygen.

During initial stabilization and pain management the patient begins to complain of increased pain. The monitor reveals the following rhythm:

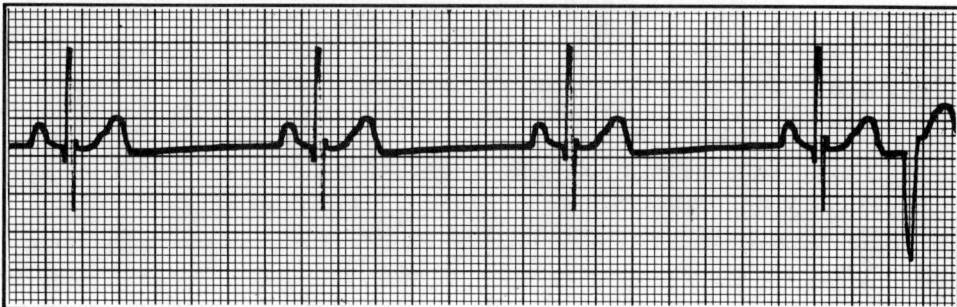

112. ECG interpretation is:

    A. Sinus rhythm with frequent multifocal PVCs.
    B. Sinus rhythm with frequent unifocal PVCs.
    C. Sinus bradycardia with frequent junctional complexes.
    D. Sinus bradycardia with ventricular escape complexes.

113. What is the most appropriate intervention at this time?

    A. Nothing—no intervention is required.
    B. Lidocaine 1 mg/kg IV bolus.
    C. Atropine 0.5 mg IV bolus.
    D. Isoproterenol titrated to a pulse rate of 60/min.

Questions 114–117 relate to the following situation:

You respond to a call for a 70-year-old female who had a syncopal episode lasting about one minute according to bystanders. She is responsive now and does not know what happened. She has a previous history of hypertension and takes some type of diuretic. She has had "palpitations" off and on for the past week. There is no evidence of tongue biting or incontinence. She denies chest pain or dyspnea and feels fine now. She is alert and has no neurologic deficit; her lungs are clear and her physical exam is unremarkable. Vital signs are pulse 90, respirations 18, BP 170/90, SpO_2 98. ECG is as follows. She is refusing medical attention.

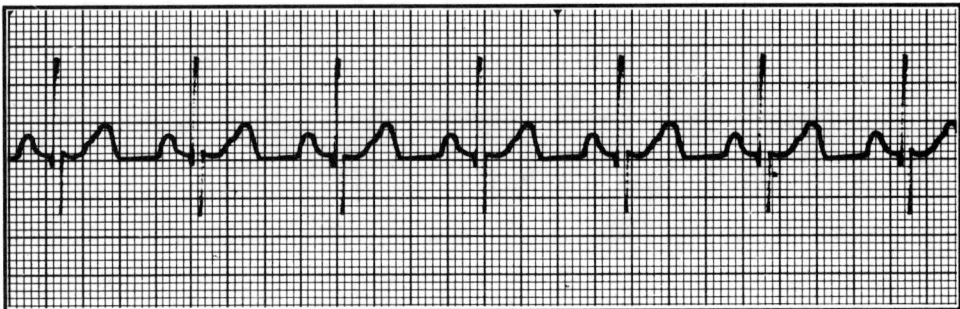

114. Your ECG interpretation is:

    A. Normal sinus rhythm.
    B. Wandering atrial pacemaker.
    C. First-degree AV block.
    D. Normal sinus rhythm with PACs.

115. The most appropriate approach to handling this situation is:

    A. Allow her to refuse medical attention and sign off.
    B. Convince her to seek attention on her own.
    C. Convince her to seek attention and triage her to a BLS unit.
    D. Convince her to seek attention and triage her as ALS.

116. You suspect which of the following conditions as the cause of syncope in this patient?

    A. Stokes-Adams syndrome.
    B. Wernicke-Korsakoff syndrome.
    C. Idiopathic seizure.
    D. Transient ischemic attack.

117. What is the most appropriate treatment for this patient?

    A. No immediate care is necessary.
    B. BLS supportive care and transportation.
    C. Oxygen therapy, IV access, and cardiac monitoring.
    D. Oxygen therapy, IV access, and 50% dextrose IV.

Questions 118–121 relate to the following situation:

You are called to the office of a 45-year-old male who had a sudden onset of shortness of breath and pounding in his chest. He has no significant medical history, and he denies chest pain. He does complain of feeling faint. His vital signs are pulse difficult to palpate at 170, respirations 30, BP 118/70, SpO$_2$ 96. He is diaphoretic and pale. ECG is as follows. There are no other positive physical findings.

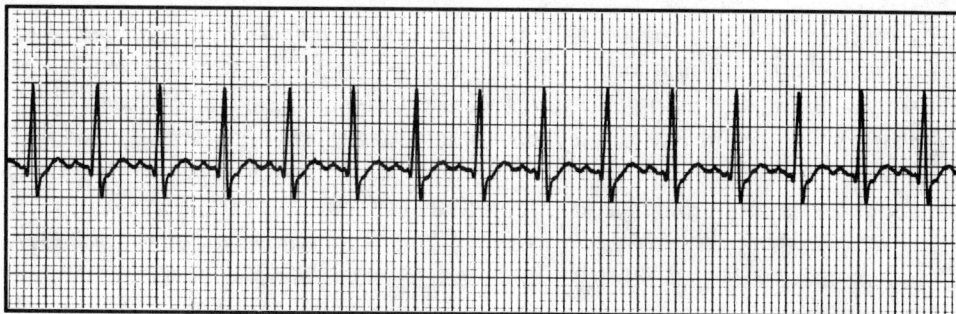

118. ECG interpretation is:

    A. Ventricular tachycardia.
    B. Supraventricular tachycardia.
    C. Paroxysmal supraventricular tachycardia.
    D. Sinus tachycardia.

119. After airway and venous access, which of the following would be the most appropriate intervention?

    A. Synchronized cardioversion.
    B. Vagal maneuvers.
    C. Verapamil or adenosine.
    D. Lidocaine.

120. Prior to the specific intervention in the preceding question, which of the following must be accomplished?

    A. Determine if equal carotid pulses and bruits are present.
    B. Determine if the patient has Wolf-Parkinson-White syndrome.
    C. Determine if the patient has allergy to lidocaine.
    D. Determine if the patient has a history of previous intubations.

121. What is one of the major side effects of the method chosen to terminate this dysrhythmia?

    A. Seizure.
    B. Hypotension.
    C. Brady-asystole.
    D. Ventricular fibrillation.

Questions 122–125 relate to the following situation:

You are called to a convenience medical care clinic to transport an 81-year-old female who walked into the facility with sudden onset of shortness of breath. She complains of chest pain, and she self-administered nitroglycerin. Her pain is a 6 on a scale of 1 to 10. She has a history of stable angina and takes nitroglycerin prn. There are fine crackles in both posterior bases, pulse irregular, respirations 32, BP 180/90, SpO_2 91. She is diaphoretic, restless, pale, and able to communicate verbally. The ECG is as follows. The clinic staff has administered nasal oxygen at 4 L/min and established an IV with D_5W. They have released the patient to you and asked you to follow your own protocols.

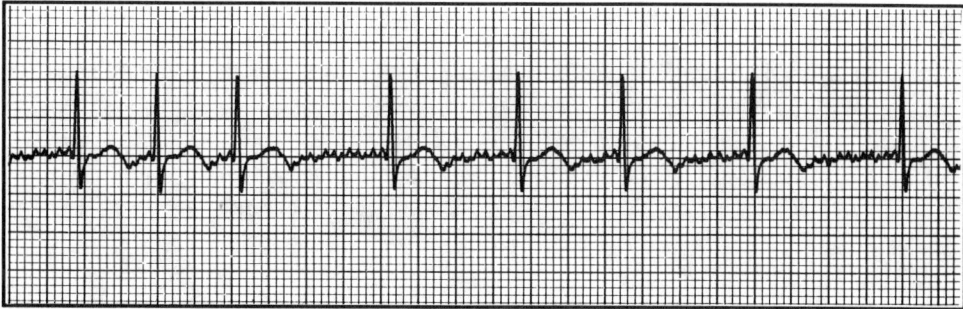

122. Your ECG interpretation is:

    A. Sinus tachycardia with frequent PACs.
    B. Supraventricular tachycardia.
    C. Atrial fibrillation.
    D. Sinus rhythm with PVCs.

123. The SpO_2 reading indicates an oxygen saturation level:

    A. Much less than 60 torr.
    B. Slightly more than 60 torr.
    C. Nearly 100 torr.
    D. Over 100 torr.

124. Which of the following is the most important initial intervention for this patient?

    A. Begin ventilation by bag-valve-mask.
    B. Perform blind nasotracheal intubation and ventilation.
    C. Administer oxygen by nonrebreathing mask at 10–15 L/min.
    D. Administer oxygen by simple face mask at 10–15 L/min.

125. What is the most appropriate initial pharmacologic intervention?

    A. Morphine 2–4 mg IV.
    B. Furosemide 40–80 mg IV.
    C. Lidocaine 100 mg IV.
    D. Verapamil 5 mg IV.

Questions 126–128 relate to the following situation:

You are called to treat a 70-year-old male who was found unresponsive by relatives. He is now verbally responsive and complains of extreme weakness and chest pressure. He has an extensive cardiac history and takes Lanoxin, nitroglycerin, and hydrochlorothiazide. He is diaphoretic and pale. Vitals are pulse weak, respirations 22, BP 86/palpation, SpO₂ 94. ECG is as follows. There are fine crackles at both posterior bases.

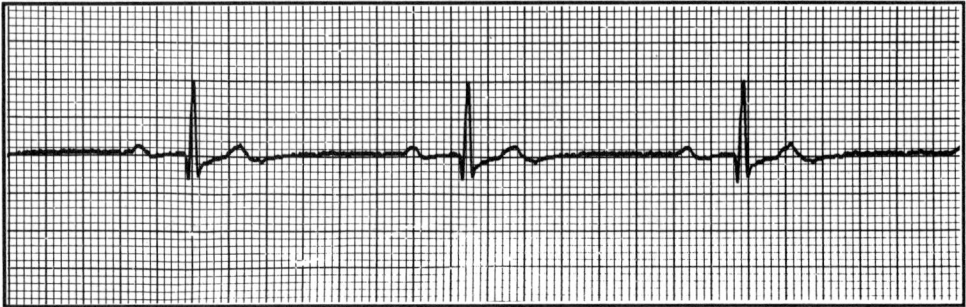

126. Your ECG interpretation is:

    A. Junctional rhythm.
    B. Complete heart block.
    C. Second-degree AV block
    D. First-degree AV block.

127. After airway management, oxygenation, and gaining IV access, what is the most appropriate initial intervention?

    A. Furosemide 40–80 mg IV.
    B. Atropine 0.5–1.0 mg IV
    C. Isoproterenol infusion titrated to a ventricular rate of 60.
    D. Dopamine 5–10 mcg/kg/min.

128. The patient still complains of chest pressure, feels very weak, is diaphoretic, and pale. His ECG is now as shown below; BP is 86/palpation. The most appropriate pharmacologic intervention is to administer:

    A. Morphine 2–4 mg IV.
    B. Atropine 0.5–1.0 mg IV.

C. Isoproterenol infusion titrated to a ventricular rate of 60.
D. Dopamine 5–10 mcg/kg/min.

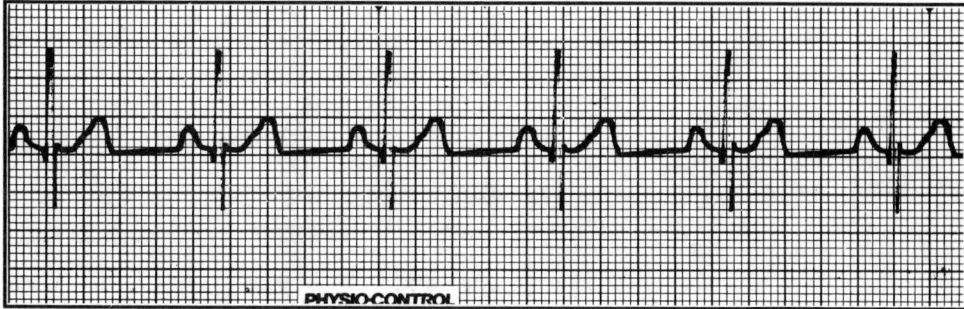

Questions 129–130 relate to the following situation:

You are called to the home of a 49-year-old male complaining of nausea and vomiting of two hours duration. He also complains of a severe headache and blurred vision. He denies any loss of consciousness, chest pain, or breathing difficulty. He has a history of hypertension and is on antihypertensive medication. He is moving all extremities; pupils are equal and react to light. Vital signs are pulse strong, respirations 26, BP 240/130, SpO$_2$ 98. His ECG is as follows:

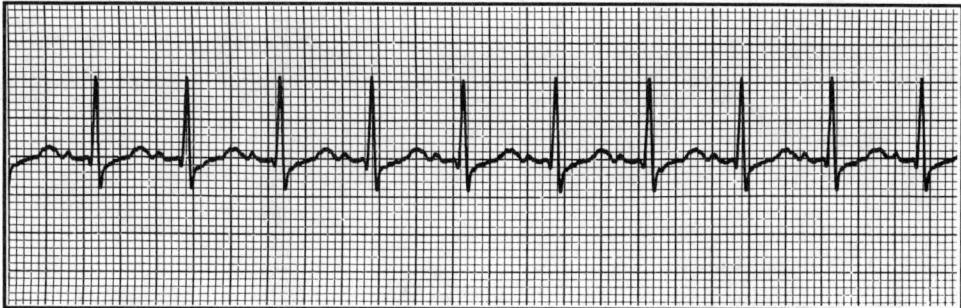

129. Your ECG interpretation is:

   A. Ventricular tachycardia.
   B. Sinus tachycardia.
   C. Supraventricular tachycardia.
   D. Normal sinus rhythm.

130. All of the following medications may be used in the treatment of this patient's presenting problem *except*:

    A. Nifedipine.
    B. Nitroglycerin.
    C. Furosemide.
    D. Verapamil.

Questions 131–132 relate to the following situation:

You are called to a nursing home to treat a 52-year-old female nursing assistant who had a sudden onset of nausea and feeling weak and faint. She has a previous history of mitral valve replacement 20 years ago and an AMI at that time. She denies chest pain or dyspnea. She takes the following medications: Coumadin, Lanoxin, and nitroglycerin prn. She is pale and diaphoretic. Her vitals are pulse 46 and very irregular, respirations 26, BP 92/30, SpO$_2$ 95. Her ECG is as follows:

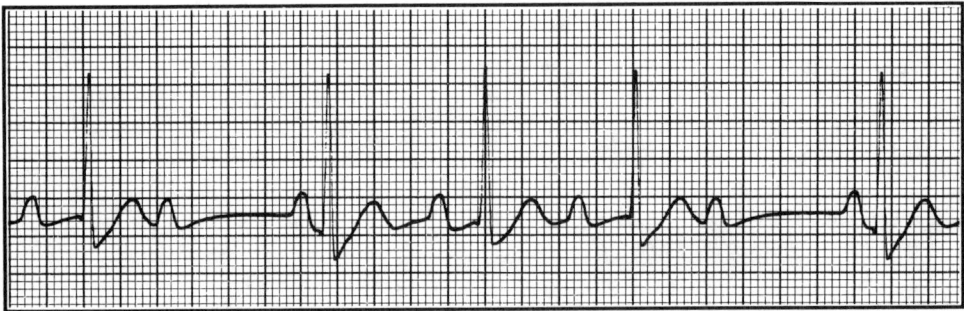

131. Your ECG interpretation is:

    A. Atrial fibrillation.
    B. Sinus bradycardia.
    C. Second-degree AV block Type I.
    D. Third-degree AV block.

132. The initial treatment for this patient includes which of the following?

    A. External pacing.
    B. Isoproterenol.
    C. Atropine.
    D. Crystalloid fluid challenge.

Endocrine System

133. You are called to a local business because a 42-year-old female collapsed while on her way to a meeting. Co-workers report she has been jumpy and irritable all day. No additional medical history is possible. A bottle of DiaBeta is found in her desk by a co-worker while you are doing the assessment. After several attempts, you find it impossible to start an IV and decide to administer:

    A. 10% dextrose SQ.
    B. Narcan 1 mg IM.
    C. Epinephrine 0.3 mg SQ.
    D. Glucagon 1 mg IM.

134. Which of the following statements concerning insulin is *incorrect*?

    A. Insulin is produced by the delta cells in the islets of Langerhans.
    B. Insulin allows glucose transport into muscle and fat cells.
    C. Insulin inhibits the process of glycogenolysis in the liver.
    D. Insulin is unnecessary for glucose transport into brain cells.

135. A transient was found lying on a park bench. Police called EMS when they were unable to rouse him. You find an unresponsive male in his mid-to-late 40s in a supine position. While securing the airway, you note an odor of ETOH. What is the first medication of choice in this situation?

    A. 50% dextrose/water.
    B. Naloxone 2 mg.
    C. Thiamine 100 mg.
    D. Either A or B are acceptable.

136. Signs and symptoms associated with a hypoglycemic reaction in the insulin-dependent diabetic result from the:

    A. Absence of glucose for brain cell function.
    B. Inadequate transport of glucose for metabolism into the cells due to lack of insulin.
    C. Inadequate synthesis of glycogen.
    D. Increased osmotic diuresis.

137. The quantity of glucose in a 50% DW preloaded syringe is:

    A. 12.5 g.
    B. 25 g.
    C. 50 g.
    D. 100 g.

138. You are called for an "unconscious female." On arrival, you are met by a teenage girl frantically waving her arms. Inside the home, you find a woman, approximately 45 years of age, lying on the sofa who responds incoherently to verbal stimuli. The girl hysterically tells you that her mother is a diabetic and that she found her this way when she came home from school. You are unable to obtain further information other than a recent history of gastroenteritis. Physical findings include: pulse 120/weak, respirations 36/deep, blood pressure 98/62. You would expect a dextrose reagent strip to show:

    A. 50.
    B. 80.
    C. 120.
    D. 200.

139. Your patient is an unconscious 19-year-old male who collapsed on the sidewalk. His skin is pale and diaphoretic; pulse is rapid and weak. The first medication of choice is:

    A. Narcan.
    B. 50% glucose.
    C. Oxygen.
    D. Either A or B.

140. Your patient is a 71-year-old male. Examination reveals poor skin turgor, hemiplegia, dry oral mucosa, and aphasia. Findings include a glucose reagent of >150 and blood pressure reading of 86/50. His pulse corresponds with the ECG:

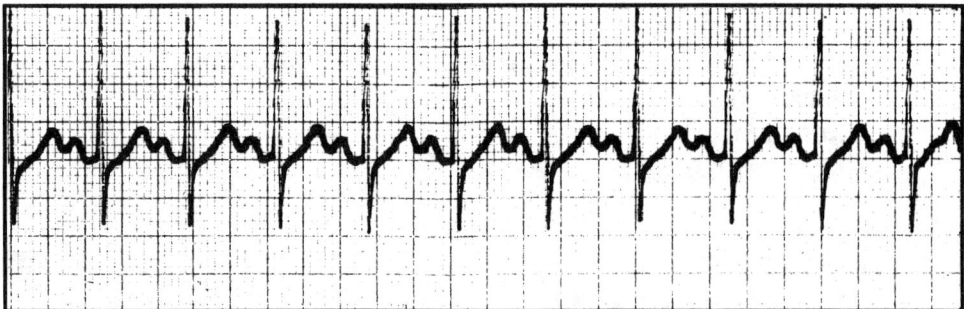

He is compliant with medication therapy which includes Glucotrol, Lanoxin, and Lasix. Management would include which of the following?

A. Crystalloid fluid resuscitation.
B. Sodium nitroprusside at 10 mcg/min.
C. Dobutamine hydrochloride drip at 2.5 mcg/min.
D. Dopamine infusion titrated to body weight and effect.

141. When administering 50% glucose by direct IV push, you must observe closely for:

A. Peripheral vasodilation.
B. Local tissue infiltration.
C. Ventricular irritability.
D. Diminished sensorium.

Nervous System

142. A 29-year-old male was involved in a motorcycle accident. He is found lying approximately 200 feet from the wreckage. His friend tells you that the patient was not wearing a helmet when he lost control of the bike and crashed. He is exhibiting decerebrate posturing and fixed, dilated pupils. You suspect injury involving the brain stem. Which of the following statements regarding the brain stem are correct? The brain stem:

(1) Is located inferior to the cerebellum.
(2) Lies anterior to the cerebrum.
(3) Includes the diencephalon and medulla.
(4) Regulates coordination and peripheral proprioception.

A. 1, 2, 3.
B. 1, 3.
C. 2, 3, 4.
D. 2, 4.

143. The nervous system is structurally divided into which parts?

A. Brain and spinal cord.
B. Afferent and efferent divisions.
C. Autonomic and involuntary subsystems.
D. Central and peripheral nervous systems.

144. Control centers for regulation of heartbeat, respirations, and blood pressure are located in which area?

   A. Cerebrum.
   B. Cerebellum.
   C. Midbrain.
   D. Medulla.

145. The crossover of nerves from the left brain to the right side of the body and from the right brain to the left side of the body occurs at the level of the:

   A. Cerebrum.
   B. Cerebellum.
   C. Midbrain.
   D. Medulla.

146. Which of the following components are quantitatively evaluated on the Glasgow Coma Scale?

   A. Sensory, motor, pupils.
   B. Motor, verbal response, LOC.
   C. Motor, verbal response, eye opening.
   D. Pupils, LOC, motor.

147. Signs of increasing intracranial pressure include which of the following?

   (1) Altered LOC.
   (2) Unequal pupils/dilated pupils.
   (3) Drop in BP, rise in pulse.
   (4) Rise in BP, drop in pulse.
   (5) Loss of peripheral pulses.

   A. 1, 2, 3.
   B. 1, 3, 4.
   C. 2, 4, 5.
   D. 1, 2, 4.

148. What mechanism causes shock in the spinal cord-injured patient?

   A. Loss of parasympathetic tone.
   B. Loss of sympathetic tone.
   C. Presence of blood in the spinal canal.
   D. Injuries to the thoracic cage.

149. You are called to a baseball game where a 9-year-old boy has been injured. A bystander noticed that the boy's left hand began to twitch, and the twitching progressed up his left arm before subsiding. The entire episode lasted about three minutes. You suspect that the patient has suffered which type of seizure?

   A. Focal motor (Jacksonian) seizure.
   B. Psychomotor seizure.
   C. Petit mal seizure.
   D. Grand mal seizure.

150. Which is the most correct statement regarding generalized motor seizures?

   A. They do not require patient transport to the hospital if the patient is known to be an epileptic.
   B. They are characterized by an altered personality state before the seizure begins.
   C. They are always associated with an aura.
   D. They may result from traumatic or medical causes.

151. Which statements best describe status epilepticus?

   (1) Management of status epilepticus is the same as management for any generalized motor seizure.
   (2) Status epilepticus is considered a serious medical emergency.
   (3) Status epilepticus may lead to serious complications.
   (4) Status epilepticus is often caused by failure to take anticonvulsant medications.
   (5) Status epilepticus cannot be effectively managed in the field.

   A. 1, 2, 4.
   B. 2, 3, 4.
   C. 1, 2, 5.
   D. 3, 4, 5.

152. What is your first intervention if you find a patient actively seizing?

   A. Place a tongue blade between the patient's teeth.
   B. Protect from injury.
   C. Administer diazepam.
   D. Restrain the patient.

153. Which of the following statements is most accurate regarding a cerebro-vascular accident (CVA)?

    A. CVA may occur in any age group.
    B. CVA occurs without prior warning.
    C. CVA results in permanent hemiplegia.
    D. CVA requires long-term hospital rehabilitation.

154. Which of the following treatment modalities are most appropriate in the field management of the patient who has suffered a CVA?

    (1) Oxygen.
    (2) Trendelenburg position.
    (3) Elevate head 15 degrees.
    (4) Hyperventilate if unresponsive.
    (5) Administer corticosteroids.

    A. 1, 2, 4.
    B. 1, 4, 5.
    C. 1, 3, 4.
    D. 1, 3, 5.

155. Which of the following statements is most correct regarding field neurologic assessment?

    A. Therapy is based on the initial Glasgow Coma score.
    B. The Glasgow Coma score is the best single predictor of survival.
    C. The field neurologic assessment provides a baseline of information.
    D. Deep tendon reflexes are an important part of the field neurologic exam.

156. Which of the following reactions does *not* occur in the brain as a result of hypoventilation in the head-injured patient?

    A. Increased $PaCO_2$.
    B. Vasodilation.
    C. Vasoconstriction.
    D. Rise in intracranial pressure.

157. You are called to the office of a 56-year-old male who experienced an episode of aphasia. When he tried to walk to his secretary's desk, his right leg did not support him resulting in a fall. On your arrival, he can stand, although somewhat unsteadily. He is able to relate these events.

The episode lasted approximately 30 minutes. Which of the following is the most likely disease process in this situation?

A. Embolic stroke.
B. Thrombotic stroke.
C. Psychomotor seizure.
D. Transient ischemic attack.

158. A 40-year-old robbery victim was shot in the frontal lobe with a small caliber weapon. Which of the following specialized functions are located in the frontal lobe?

(1) Speech.
(2) Vision.
(3) Personality.
(4) Balance and coordination.
(5) Motor.

A. 1, 3.
B. 2, 4.
C. 4, 5.
D. 3, 5.

159. Which of the following body systems dominates during the acute stress response?

A. Parasympathetic nervous system.
B. Sympathetic nervous system.
C. Central nervous system.
D. Peripheral nervous system.

160. Which of the following drugs is *not* considered appropriate in the field management of a coma?

A. Sodium bicarbonate.
B. Naloxone.
C. Thiamine.
D. Dexamethasone.

161. You respond to the bus station on a "man down." On arrival, you find a male in his mid-40s who appears to be having a generalized major motor seizure. No history is available. Seizure activity stops briefly, but before the patient regains consciousness, generalized seizure activity

resumes. Which of the following would be included in the initial management of this patient?

(1) High flow oxygen by bag-valve-mask.
(2) Endotracheal intubation.
(3) Diazepam 5–10 mg IV.
(4) Dextrose 50%, 25 g IV push.
(5) Mannitol 25 g IV over 30 minutes.

A. 1, 3, 4.
B. 1, 2, 3.
C. 1, 2, 3, 4.
D. 1, 3, 4, 5.

Acute Abdomen

162. A 27-year-old male experienced sudden onset of chest pain and dyspnea while receiving home hemodialysis. You find the patient with hemodi-alysis in progress via a left arm fistula. As you begin your assessment, he takes a deep breath and coughs. A few gasping respirations are followed by respiratory arrest. Due to his condition you must immediately:

A. Prepare him for endotracheal intubation.
B. Place him in a left, lateral recumbent position.
C. Prepare for a quick look and possible defibrillation.
D. Apply a tourniquet to his left arm above the fistula.

163. You are called to the home of a 45-year-old female complaining of severe RUQ pain that started approximately two hours ago. Physical examination reveals an overweight patient with RUQ guarding and tenderness. She complains of extreme nausea and begins to vomit. There is no previous history of similar episodes, pertinent past medical history, known allergies, or current medications. You would suspect:

A. Perforated duodenal ulcer.
B. Acute peptic ulcer.
C. Cholecystitis.
D. Hepatitis.

164. Your patient is a 67-year-old male. He is complaining of severe LLQ pain and nausea. There is no additional medical history. His problem is most likely due to:

A. Appendicitis.
B. Cholecystitis.
C. Diverticulitis.
D. Duodenal ulcer.

165. Mr. Byers is a 26-year-old male complaining of severe right flank pain. Preparing for transport is difficult because he is extremely restless and will not lie still. He has had hematuria for the past two days. Vital signs are P 100/regular, R 24/unlabored, BP 156/86. You suspect:

A. Acute appendicitis.
B. Ruptured diverticulum.
C. Renal calculus with obstruction.
D. Perforated viscus with peritonitis.

166. Sara is a 17-year-old female complaining of severe LLQ pain. Assessment of the patient should proceed in which of the following sequences?

A. RLQ to RUQ to LUQ to LLQ.
B. RUQ to RLQ to LLQ to LUQ.
C. LLQ to LUQ to RUQ to RLQ.
D. LUQ to RUQ to RLQ to LLQ.

167. Your patient is a 56-year-old female. She is complaining of abdominal pain that began two hours before she called EMS. Your assessment reveals a pulsating mass to the left of the umbilicus. You suspect which condition?

A. Peritonitis.
B. Abdominal aortic aneurysm.
C. Ruptured spleen.
D. Appendicitis.

168. A 14-year-old male presents with an acute onset of atraumatic testicular pain and edema. You suspect which condition?

A. Epididymitis.
B. Torsion.
C. Orchitis.
D. Prostatitis.

169. You are called to treat a 39-year-old female after she collapsed at a service station. She is unresponsive. She has a patent airway with rapid, shallow respirations, and a weak, rapid carotid pulse. There is no evidence of trauma or external hemorrhage. No one at the scene is able to provide additional information. Examination reveals a clamped clear catheter protruding from the midline at the periumbilical region. Her past medical history could include which of the following?

    A. Continuous ambulatory peritoneal dialysis (CAPD).
    B. End-stage renal disease (ESRD).
    C. Insulin-dependent diabetes mellitus (IDDM).
    D. All of the above.

170. A 52-year-old male, with a history of acute myocardial infarction (AMI) two weeks ago, is complaining of nonradiating epigastric pain and nausea. History of present illness includes hematemesis and melena for two days. He is pale, cool, and diaphoretic with the following vital signs: P 136/weak, R 24/shallow, BP 96/70. Treatment could include all of the following *except*:

    A. Fluid resuscitation.
    B. Oxygen per cannula.
    C. PASG inflation.
    D. Dopamine infusion.

171. A 29-year-old female completed hemodialysis and was awaiting a ride home when she collapsed in front of the Dialysis Center. Upon arrival, you find her on an exam table. She is complaining of dizziness and slight nausea. Her skin is pale, cool, and clammy. Her pulse is 122/weak, respirations 24/shallow, BP 80/40. The left forearm fistula site has a thrill and bruit present. Care for this patient would include:

    A. Fluid resuscitation with lactated Ringer's.
    B. Oxygen administration and ECG monitoring.
    C. IV of D_5W KVO and dopamine titrated to effect.
    D. Both A and B.

Anaphylaxis

172. In a sensitized individual, contact with an antigen produces which one of the following reactions?

A. Production of antibodies to the specific antigen.
B. Attachment of antibodies to mast cells.
C. Release of histamine and heparin from antibodies.
D. Release of histamine and heparin from mast cells.

173. The maximum initial adult dose of the antihistamine indicated in the treatment of anaphylaxis is:

A. 0.5 mg.
B. 50 mg.
C. 50 mg/kg/min.
D. 500 mg.

174. Your patient is a 36-year-old male who has been taking penicillin for a throat infection. He is complaining of dyspnea and pharyngeal pruritus. His pulse is 140 and weak, respirations 36 and labored, BP 100/70. Your orders include the administration of aminophylline because it will:

A. Increase the cardiac output and tissue perfusion.
B. Suppress the body's inflammatory response.
C. Increase peripheral vascular resistance.
D. Promote bronchial dilatation.

175. When administering parenteral Benadryl to an adult, what is the preferred route?

A. SQ.
B. Rapid IV push.
C. Deep IM.
D. Slow IV drip infusion.

Toxicology, Alcohol and Drug Abuse

176. You are called to a home where a 3-year-old boy has been found unconscious. The patient has burns surrounding his mouth and in the oral cavity. There is a container of a concentrated commercial liquid drain opener lying next to the patient. He is breathing, pulse is 100, and blood pressure is 90/40. Which of the following actions is *not* appropriate in the management of this patient?

A. Provide a patent airway.
B. Induce vomiting with syrup of ipecac.

    C. Start an IV with D₅W.

    D. Rapid transport to the hospital.

177. A farmer was working with a herbicide containing paraquat. After visiting with another farmer, he forgot he had put a portion of the substance in a cup. He then inadvertently consumed a small amount. In this situation, it is contraindicated to administer:

    A. IV furosemide.

    B. Supplemental oxygen.

    C. Crystalloid IV fluids.

    D. Mannitol solutions.

178. Mrs. Smith has been prescribed diazepam for her anxiety states. At first, she took 5-mg tablets prn. Now she finds that 10 mg are needed to produce the same effect. This process is called:

    A. Psychologic dependence.

    B. Tolerance.

    C. Physical dependence.

    D. Addiction.

179. Your unit has responded to a local electroplating factory where you find a 24-year-old male who became acutely ill. He is responsive to verbal stimulus with a pulse of 130 and respiratory rate of 30/shallow. During the secondary assessment, you note twitching and spasms of the extremities. Co-workers said he was working alone in an isolated location before staggering into their area. During venipuncture, you note that his blood is markedly bright red. The first drug of choice is:

    A. Oxygen.

    B. 50% dextrose in water.

    C. Amyl nitrite.

    D. Sodium thiosulfate.

180. About eight hours before calling EMS, an 18-year-old female overdosed because she had an argument with her mother. She is complaining of tinnitus, nausea, and faintness. Assessment reveals hot and dry skin, tachypnea, hyperpnea, and tachycardia. After establishing a patent airway, administering oxygen, and starting an IV, you would consider which of the following medications?

A. Activated charcoal.
B. Sodium bicarbonate.
C. Syrup of ipecac.
D. None of the above is necessary because the amount taken is not potentially dangerous.

181. A 21-year-old female is complaining of chills, fever, nausea, and vomiting that began yesterday. She contacted EMS because the rash she had on her left foot "turned black and began hurting real bad." She said she was "afraid of blood poisoning" when the recent symptoms started. Physical examination of the left foot reveals a bull's eye lesion with a considerable area of necrosis. You suspect envenomization by a:

A. Scorpion.
B. Brown recluse spider.
C. Pit viper.
D. Black widow spider.

182. You are treating a 36-year-old female who ingested approximately twenty 75-mg imipramine tablets. You have intubated the trachea and started an IV. The ECG shows the following:

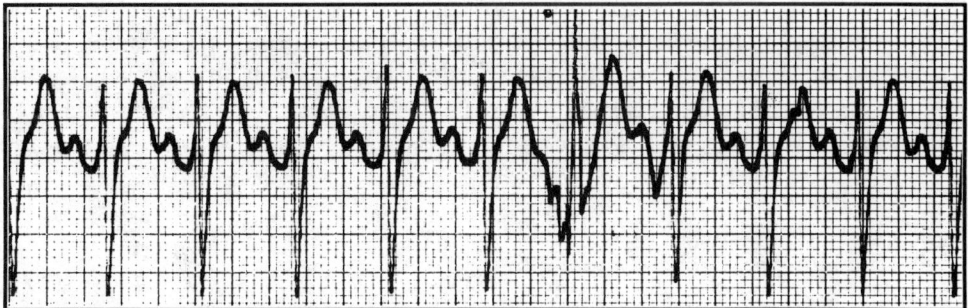

Initial management of this dysrhythmia requires:

A. Sodium bicarbonate.
B. Physostigmine.
C. Quinidine.
D. None of the above.

183. You are called to a garden nursery to treat a 32-year-old male who suddenly became ill while spraying an insecticide. He is disoriented, the skin is pale and moist, and he is salivating excessively. Vital signs are pulse corresponds to the ECG, respirations 24, BP 138/80. Pupils are slightly constricted. Slight seizure activity is noted in the left arm. What is the initial dosage of the first parenteral drug of choice for this patient?

A. 0.01 ml/kg up to 0.5 ml.
B. 0.4 mg.
C. 2.0 mg.
D. 25 g in a 50% solution.

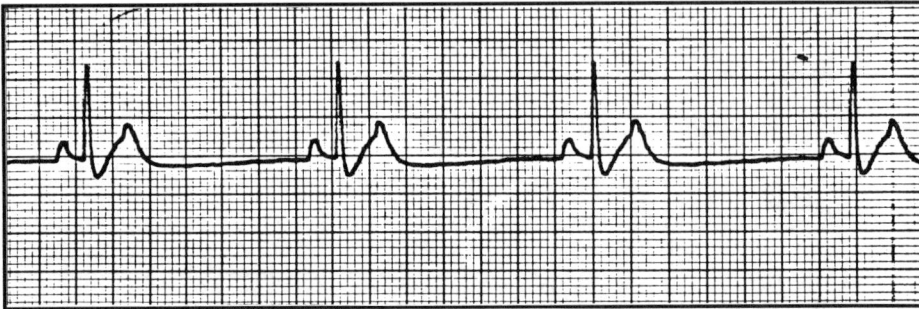

184. A 24-year-old woman, who broke her engagement, is found unconscious clutching an unmarked bottle containing one bright red capsule. On examination, you find her responsive to painful stimuli with a few slurred mumbles. Pulse is 100/regular, respirations 8/minute and shallow, BP 90/70. Her skin is cool and dry. Pupils are widely dilated and poorly reactive. You suspect she has taken:

A. Cocaine.
B. Heroin.
C. Seconal.
D. Phencyclidine.

185. A 12-year-old female was bitten by a snake while hiking in wooded terrain. She experienced instantaneous pain with edema at the site of the injury. Now, approximately one hour later, she is complaining of nausea and dizziness. Pulse is 120/min, respirations 32/min and shallow, BP 80/20. The hospital is approximately five minutes away. Management of this patient could include all of the following *except:*

A. Cold application.
B. Limb immobilization.
C. Crystalloid fluids IV.
D. Constricting band above the wound.

186. Your patient is an automotive mechanic who is complaining of a throbbing headache and dizziness. While at the scene, ten other mechanics begin to report nausea and inability to concentrate. You suspect toxicity due to inhalation of:

A. Chlorine.
B. Carbon monoxide.
C. Ammonia.
D. Aromatic benzenes.

187. All of the following statements are true about the alcohol withdrawal syndrome *except*:

A. Tremulousness is a common finding.
B. DTs usually occur one week after the last drink.
C. Seizures tend to occur early in the withdrawal phase.
D. Physical effects occur as the blood alcohol level reaches zero.

188. Your patient is a "regular" with a known history of chronic alcoholism. The police called because they found him unresponsive. Next to him, your partner finds a container labeled "Wood Alcohol." What is the antidote indicated in this situation?

A. Activated charcoal.
B. Syrup of ipecac.
C. Ethylene glycol.
D. Ethanol.

Infectious Diseases

189. HIV infects which of the following?

A. T-helper lymphocytes.
B. T-suppressor lymphocytes.
C. B lymphocytes.
D. Circulating antibodies.

190. A 9-month-old was unresponsive when his parents checked him before going to bed. On your arrival, the mother is frantically waving directions to the house. Initial examination of the infant reveals nuchal rigidity and generalized petechiae on the body. You suspect:

    A. Rubella.
    B. Rheumatic fever.
    C. Meningococcal meningitis.
    D. Reye's syndrome with encephalopathy.

191. Which of the following modes of transmission can potentially constitute a true exposure to the HIV virus?

    A. Blood contact.
    B. Saliva contact.
    C. Skin contact.
    D. Droplets in the air.

192. A condition that is characterized by a positive HIV, with the presence of a disease indicative of an underlying cellular immune deficiency in a person with no known cause for such a deficiency defines:

    A. ARC.
    B. AIDS.
    C. Immunodeficiency.
    D. All of the above.

193. Leslie Neal is a 19-year-old male complaining of pleuritic chest pain associated with productive cough, fever, night sweats, and abdominal pain for eight days. He appears thin and emaciated. When asked why he called EMS today, he says his doctor gave him "some medicine that isn't doing any good." In addition to acetaminophen for fever, he also takes isoniazid. You would recognize that Mr. Neal is being treated for:

    A. Pneumonia.
    B. Pneumocystis.
    C. Tuberculosis.
    D. Immune deficiency.

194. You are treating a patient who has herpes zoster. Which of the following statements is *not* true about this condition?

A. There is no known cure for this disease.
B. Patients with this condition have a past history of chickenpox.
C. Skin eruptions follow a cranial or spinal nerve tract.
D. Communicability is low after the blisters have erupted.

195. While rendering care to a patient, she informs you that she is being treated for delta hepatitis. You can assume her medical history includes:

A. Hepatitis A (HAV).
B. Hepatitis B (HBV).
C. Hepatitis C (HCV).
D. Hepatitis NANB.

196. What is the best disinfectant for effectively disinfecting the ambulance between calls?

A. Isopropyl alcohol.
B. Tuberculocidal agent.
C. Betadine iodine solution.
D. 1:100 bleach/water solution.

197. A 49-year-old female presents with malaise, abdominal pain, and anorexia. She states that she thought she had the flu but has gotten worse over the past several days. She called EMS because she was afraid to drive to the hospital because she was weak. Physical examination is essentially unremarkable except for scleral icterus. There is no past medical history. You assume this patient's problem is due to:

A. Hepatitis A.
B. An acute abdomen.
C. Salmonella infection.
D. Gastroenteritis.

Environmental Injuries

198. Your ALS unit has been on stand-by at an underwater diving (SCUBA) exhibition. Two divers run to your location after a 27-year-old novice rapidly ascended. You find the patient responds meaningfully to verbal stimuli and has a patent airway. Physical examination reveals abnormal

heart sounds and mild cyanosis. His pulse is 130/irregular, respirations 28/labored, and BP is 80/66. When he attempts to describe his chest pain, you note his voice is hoarse. You suspect this patient has:

A. Hemopericardium.
B. Tension pneumothorax.
C. Pneumomediastinum.
D. Venous air embolism.

199. You respond to a "man down" in a dry cleaning establishment. A 33-year-old pressman collapsed after complaining of weakness and nausea. On arrival, you find that the patient has regained consciousness. He is pale, cool, and clammy and has a thready pulse. You would suspect:

A. Heat exhaustion.
B. Heat cramps.
C. Heat stroke.
D. Any of the above could apply.

200. A 17-year-old male dove into a lake from a rock. When he did not surface immediately, one of his friends located and extricated him from the water. The best method(s) for opening this patient's airway is/are:

A. Modified jaw thrust.
B. Head-tilt with chin-lift.
C. Triple airway maneuver.
D. Either A or C is acceptable.

201. An after-drop core temperature decrease can result in:

A. Acidosis.
B. Ventricular fibrillation.
C. Increased metabolic demands.
D. Both A and B.

202. A 59-year-old female was found in her unheated apartment during a neighborhood check in early February. Primary assessment reveals a patent airway, shallow respirations at 4/min, and a weak carotid pulse. The quick look reveals the following:

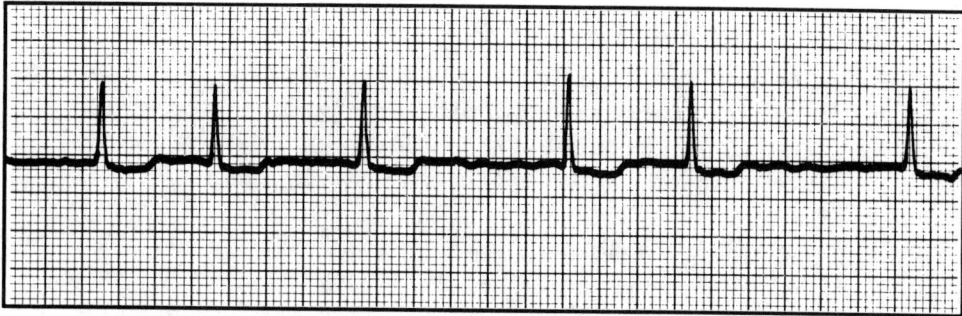

What is your initial intervention?

A. Assist ventilations with bag-valve-mask and 100% oxygen.
B. Intubate the trachea and provide O_2 with a bag-valve device.
C. Transport the patient immediately with extreme caution.
D. Start an IV of 5% DW and contact the base station for orders.

203. Rewarming the hypothermic patient is best accomplished by the application of heat to all of the following areas *except*:

A. Lateral chest.
B. Extremities.
C. Groin.
D. Head.

204. A 32-year-old male was involved in a single-vehicle accident during a blizzard. He was pinned in the vehicle for six hours prior to being found. After extricating him, you note the following ECG:

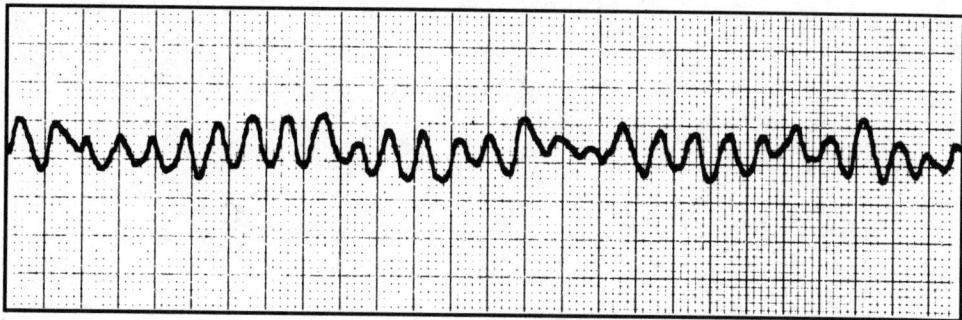

Which management technique is indicated in the care of this patient?

A. Lidocaine 1 mg/kg initially repeating 0.5 mg/kg q 5 minutes prn.
B. Defibrillation once at 360J until core temperature is measured.
C. Endotracheal intubation and ventilation with oxygen.
D. Rewarming if the scene-to-hospital ETA <10 minutes.

205. A mother left her sleeping 3-year-old in a locked car with the windows rolled up on a summer day while she "ran into the grocery store to pick up a few things." When she returned, the child was limp and unresponsive. You find the baby is hot, flushed, and dry with a full/bounding pulse. After applying cold packs, you notice the baby is shivering. Why should you discontinue the cooling efforts?

A. You can put the patient into a state of shock.
B. Shivering indicates you are dangerously close to overcooling the patient.
C. Shivering indicates a chemical imbalance.
D. Shivering is the body's mechanism for producing heat.

206. Your unit has responded to a nuclear reactor plant. The company officials usher you into the first aid station where a worker has showered following an incident in the reactor area. What must you remember in this situation?

(1) Because neutrons are usually present only near a reactor core, they are not normally a problem for paramedics.
(2) Gamma rays cause indirect damage by causing internal tissue to emit Alpha and/or Beta particles.
(3) Alpha particles can produce harmful effects if inhaled or ingested.
(4) Beta particles are lower energy than Alpha particles.

A. 1, 2, 3.
B. 1, 2, 4.
C. 2, 3.
D. 3, 4.

207. Victims of cold water near-drowning have a higher probability of survival due to what phenomenon?

A. Decreased metabolism.
B. Laryngospasm.
C. Diving reflex.
D. Hypothermia.

Geriatrics/Gerontology

208. Your patient is an 84-year-old male whose son called EMS because he "wouldn't get out of his chair." You find the patient lying on a recliner in the den. When you attempt to question him, you note his speech is incomprehensible. He appears angry as he attempts to converse with you. Examination reveals left hemiparesis and ptosis. En route, his speech begins to clear and the paresis becomes less apparent. You suspect:

    A. CVA.
    B. AMI.
    C. DKA.
    D. TIA.

209. Mrs. Telek is a 75-year-old female who called EMS because she began to experience severe dyspnea the preceding night. Physical examination reveals bilateral JVD at 45°, 4+ peripheral edema, and bilateral rales. Which of the following findings is *least* significant?

    A. JVD at 45°.
    B. Severe dyspnea.
    C. Peripheral edema.
    D. Duration of symptoms.

210. Mrs. Taylor, a normally active 89-year-old, was involved in a minor auto accident earlier in which she sustained a laceration to her upper lip and minor contusions to her chest and both arms. She was seen, treated, and released from the Emergency Department. During the night, her daughter called because Mrs. Taylor was incoherent, lethargic, and incontinent of urine. You find her lying in bed as described by the daughter. She responds to verbal stimuli but is disoriented and drifts back to sleep easily. What do you suspect?

    A. Subdural hematoma due to the accident which has slowly developed since her release from the hospital.
    B. Myocardial contusion with possible cardiogenic shock because she had bruises on her chest.
    C. Cerebrovascular accident that is unrelated to the automobile accident.
    D. Nothing. This is not an uncommon side effect of a minor head injury in an elderly patient.

211. Which of the following statements about the aging process is *not* true?

    A. The left ventricle hypertrophies up to 45%.
    B. The maximum breathing capacity decreases by 60%.
    C. There is a 15% reduction in nerve conduction velocity.
    D. There is a decrease in the total body fat of 15 to 30%.

212. Your patient is an 88-year-old female. Physical examination of both ankles reveals puffiness. There is no neck vein distention or liver engorgement. She is not acutely distressed and denies chest pain or dyspnea. The clinical picture is most likely due to:

    A. Dependent edema.
    B. Right-sided ventricular failure.
    C. Pulmonary edema.
    D. Congestive heart failure.

213. Mr. Fleming is a 73-year-old male complaining of nausea, photophobia, and paresthesia. His pulse is 80 and regular, respirations are 26 and slightly shallow, BP is 220/160. He is not currently taking any medications. The past medical history is negative. Other signs associated with his condition could include all of the following *except*:

    A. Hemiparesis.
    B. Disorientation.
    C. Staggered gait.
    D. Quadriplegia.

214. Mr. Darnell is a 66-year-old male complaining of heaviness in his chest which has persisted for one hour and increasing dyspnea. He has a history of emphysema and "heart trouble." Medications include a "heart pill" and a "water pill." R is 26, BP 124/70. Auscultation of the chest reveals bibasilar rales. His ECG is as follows:

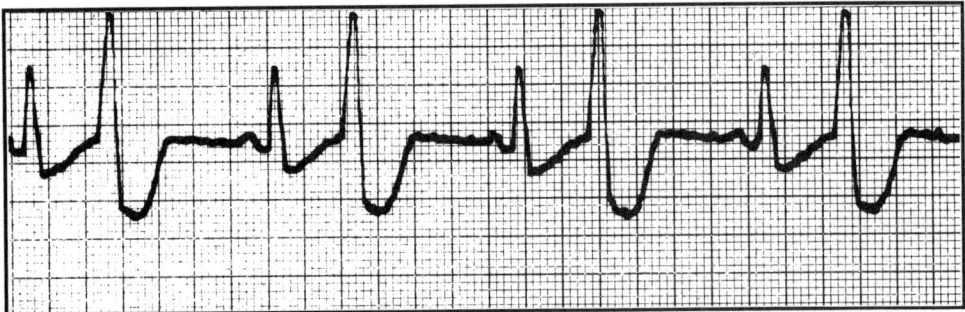

What is the initial dose of the first parenteral medication of choice in this situation?

A. 0.5 mg/kg.
B. 1.0 mg/kg.
C. 5 mcg/kg/min.
D. 20 mg/min.

215. You suspect Mr. Rich, an 88-year-old male, has a lower respiratory infection. Which of the following signs is unreliable to rule out the presence of an infectious process?

A. Poor turgor.
B. Cool, dry skin.
C. Exertional dyspnea.
D. Diffuse bilateral rales.

216. Mr. H. Moberly, an 82-year-old nursing-home resident, is to be transported to the Emergency Department because he experienced a sudden onset of confusion. All of the following could result in acute organic brain syndrome (OBS) *except*:

A. Electrolyte abnormalities.
B. Expansion of a brain tumor.
C. Alzheimer's disease.
D. Subdural hematoma.

217. You are treating a conscious 83-year-old female who, less than one hour prior to your arrival, ingested approximately thirty 50-mg amitriptyline tablets after attending her husband's funeral. Treatment of this patient could include all of the following *except*:

A. Sodium bicarbonate.
B. Induction of emesis.
C. Tracheal intubation.
D. Hyperventilation with oxygen.

218. You respond to a call on a hot, humid summer day. Your patient is a 71-year-old male who collapsed on a front lawn. Bystanders inform you that he was mowing the grass when he suddenly collapsed. Physical examination reveals dilated pupils, hot/dry skin, and a weak/thready pulse. What IV therapy is indicated in this situation?

A. 5% DW wide open.
B. 0.9 NaCl wide open.
C. 0.45 NaCl KVO.
D. D_5/0.2 NaCl KVO.

Pediatrics

219. The control of bleeding for a child with unilateral epistaxis is initially accomplished by:

A. Use of a hemostat.
B. Application of ice.
C. Packing the nose with gauze.
D. Pinching the nostrils together.

220. Following injury or accident, the young child's greatest fear is most likely:

A. Pain.
B. Separation from parents.
C. Needles.
D. The sight of blood.

221. Your basic approach to the noncritically ill or injured child will depend on which of the following?

A. The nature of the illness or injury.
B. The age of the patient.
C. The presence of the parents.
D. The environment in which you are working.

222. In a 6-month-old patient, which of the following clinical findings is most likely to be significant of a serious illness?

A. Vomiting twice.
B. Fever of 103°F rectally.
C. Pulsating anterior fontanelle.
D. Nuchal rigidity.

223. What is the most common cardiac response to hypoxia in the infant?

A. Tachycardia.
B. Bradycardia.
C. Premature ventricular contractions.
D. Premature atrial contractions.

224. Chronic bronchoconstriction that results in edema, congestion, and wheezing is termed:

A. Croup.
B. Asthma.
C. Bronchiolitis.
D. Epiglottitis.

225. You are called to see a 3-year-old child suffering from an acute asthmatic attack. The most appropriate treatment for this child would include:

A. Oxygen, IV of D5W, epinephrine 1:10,000 IV, and possibly amino-phylline IV.
B. Oxygen and albuterol via nebulizer.
C. IV of D5W and epinephrine 1:1000 SQ.
D. Epinephrine 1:1000 SQ and aminophylline IV.

226. What is the correct dosage of epinephrine 1:1000 for a 3-year-old child who weighs 15 kg?

A. 0.5 ml.
B. 0.10 ml.
C. 0.15 ml.
D. 0.25 ml.

227. Management of laryngotracheobronchitis most commonly consists of:

A. Endotracheal intubation.
B. Subcutaneous epinephrine 0.01 ml/kg.
C. Nebulized racemic epinephrine.
D. Administration of humidified air.

228. You are called to see a 6-month-old patient who has had nasal conges-tion and a cough for several days, and who now appears pale and list-less. The mother states that she has just taken the child's temperature and it is 101°F. Respiratory rate is 60/min. On chest auscultation, rales and wheezes are heard over both lung fields. You suspect this patient most likely has:

A. Asthma.
B. Croup.
C. Bronchiolitis.
D. Pneumonia.

229. Epiglottitis is an emergency situation that can be confused with croup. Which of the following most accurately depicts epiglottitis?

A. Child usually over 4, pain on swallowing, drooling, and high temperature.
B. Child usually under 4, sore throat, anorexia, and high temperature.
C. Child usually over 4, anorexia, drooling, and whooping sound on inspiration.
D. Child usually under 4, pain on swallowing, high temperature, and a high-pitched squeaking sound on inspiration.

230. When transporting a child with respiratory problems, the paramedic should administer oxygen and:

A. Place the child in a supine position.
B. Place the child in a semi-Fowler's position.
C. Place the child in a high-Fowler's position.
D. Allow the child to assume a position of comfort.

231. Which of the following statements is true concerning cardiac dysrhythmias in the otherwise healthy pediatric patient?

A. Anemia frequently results in sinus bradycardia.
B. Children usually tolerate dysrhythmias better than adults.
C. Occasional PVCs are uncommon in children.
D. Paroxysmal ventricular tachycardia requires prompt intervention.

232. What is the leading cause of death in children over 3 years of age?

A. Congenital disorders.
B. Seizures.
C. Trauma.
D. Meningitis.

233. Which of the following conditions is more likely to cause seizures in a child than in an adult?

A. Head injury.
B. Toxic ingestion.
C. Elevated temperature.
D. Hypoxia.

234. Typical autopsy findings on a victim of SIDS include which of the following?

    (1) Intrathoracic petechiae.
    (2) Pulmonary congestion.
    (3) Pneumonia.
    (4) Aspiration of gastric contents.
    (5) Septicemia.

    A. 1, 2, 3.
    B. 1, 3, 4.
    C. 2, 3, 5.
    D. 1, 2, 4.

235. Which of the following statements about SIDS is most correct?

    A. SIDS can be prevented.
    B. The cause of SIDS is unknown.
    C. SIDS is the result of child abuse.
    D. SIDS is the result of suffocation from bed clothes.

236. Which of the following injuries would you *least* suspect to have occurred as a result of child abuse?

    A. Bruises in varying stages of healing.
    B. Burns.
    C. A 3/4-inch laceration under the chin.
    D. Multiple fractures.

237. Which of the following factors is *not* a common theme in the dynamics of child abuse?

    A. The family and/or abuser are isolated with few resources.
    B. The abusive parent has low self-esteem.
    C. The abusive parent has a low education level.
    D. Expectations of the child are unrealistic.

238. Which of the following is the *least* common cause of cardiopulmonary arrest in children?

    A. Primary cardiac problems.
    B. Airway obstruction.
    C. CNS depression or injury.
    D. Near-drowning.

239. Cardiac compressions for pediatric patients during cardiopulmonary resuscitation should be performed at a rate of:

    A. 60 per minute.
    B. 80–100 per minute.
    C. 110–120 per minute.
    D. 140 per minute.

240. Which of the following techniques is *not* an acceptable method of managing an obstructed airway in an infant?

    A. Back blows.
    B. Chest thrusts.
    C. Visualization of the upper airway.
    D. Abdominal thrusts.

241. Your patient is a 15-pound, 6-month-old child found in cardiopulmonary arrest following an accidental electrical injury. Quick-look paddles show ventricular fibrillation. To defibrillate, which dose will you select initially?

    A. 1 joule/kg.
    B. 2 joules/kg.
    C. 6 joules/kg.
    D. 10 joules/kg.

242. To aid in the conversion of ventricular fibrillation in the patient in the preceding question, the paramedic decides to administer epinephrine. What is the correct dosage for this patient?

    A. 0.10 ml/kg 1:1000 solution.
    B. 0.10 ml/kg 1:10,000 solution.
    C. 0.5 ml/kg 1:10,000 solution.
    D. 1.0 ml/kg 1:10,000 solution.

243. Which of the following would be a correct single dosage of atropine for a 33-pound child?

    A. 0.05 mg.
    B. 0.06 mg.
    C. 0.2 mg.
    D. 1.0 mg.

244. Which of the following is *not* a relatively common cause of upper airway obstruction in children?

    A. Bronchiolitis.
    B. Laryngotracheobronchitis.
    C. Epiglottitis.
    D. Foreign body.

245. It is especially important to select a blood pressure cuff of the correct size to obtain an accurate reading in the pediatric patient. The appropriate size should cover what percentage of the upper arm?

    A. One-third.
    B. One-half.
    C. Two-thirds.
    D. Three-fourths.

246. Which of the following is the correct bolus dose of intravenous fluids to correct shock in the pediatric patient?

    A. 1 ml/kg.
    B. 10 ml/kg.
    C. 20 ml/kg.
    D. 100 ml/kg.

247. Cuffed endotracheal tubes can generally be used in children over which age?

    A. 4 years.
    B. 8 years.
    C. 12 years.
    D. 15 years.

248. Which of the following considerations in infant anatomy are important to airway management?

   A. The glottis is lower in the neck than in the adult.
   B. The glottis is higher in the neck than in the adult.
   C. The tongue is smaller in proportion to related structures than in the adult.
   D. The infant's vocal cords slant downward.

249. Which of the following airway adjuncts/techniques are appropriate for use in the young child in the field?

   (1) Esophageal obturator airway.
   (2) Nasotracheal intubation.
   (3) Endotracheal intubation.
   (4) Surgical cricothyrotomy.
   (5) Oxygen-powered breathing device.

   A. 3
   B. 2, 3.
   C. 1, 3, 4.
   D. 1, 3, 4, 5.

250. The purposes of a pediatric IV calibrated volume set include:

   (1) Delivery of small, measured quantities of fluid.
   (2) Administration of intravenous medication in a measured quantity of fluid.
   (3) Prevention of runaway IVs.
   (4) Filtration of IV fluids.

   A. 1, 2.
   B. 2, 3.
   C. 1, 2, 3.
   D. 1, 2, 3, 4.

251. The preferred site for intraosseous cannulation is the:

   A. Femur.
   B. Fibula.
   C. Humerus.
   D. Tibia.

252. The approach to the pediatric patient varies depending on the age of the child. Which of the following is *not* an appropriate technique in managing a noncritically ill or injured preschooler who requires placement of an IV line?

    A. Telling the child that starting the IV will hurt.
    B. Asking the parent to assist you.
    C. Explaining to the child what you are doing.
    D. Telling the child to be brave and not cry.

253. Which of the following statements is most correct concerning the pediatric patient?

    A. In hypovolemia, a drop in blood pressure occurs sooner in the child than the adult.
    B. Supine blood pressure may remain normal with a blood loss of 20–25%.
    C. Orthostatic vital signs should not be utilized when evaluating blood loss.
    D. Delayed capillary refill is a late indicator of volume depletion.

254. Which of the following statements is most correct regarding CPR for the pediatric patient?

    A. The compression-ventilation ratio is 15:1 for one-rescuer CPR.
    B. The compression-ventilation ratio is 5:1 for one-rescuer CPR.
    C. Ventilations should be delivered at a rate of 30/minute for one-rescuer CPR.
    D. Ventilations must be interposed between compressions without a pause.

255. A 1-year-old pediatric patient was found in cardiac arrest from drowning. Following 10 minutes of CPR, you decide to administer sodium bicarbonate. The patient weighs approximately 26 pounds. What dosage would you administer?

    A. 1.2 mEq.
    B. 6 mEq.
    C. 12 mEq.
    D. 24 mEq.

256. Which of the following heart rates defines the cut-off between normal sinus rhythm and bradycardia in the infant?

   A. 60 beats/min.
   B. 80 beats/min.
   C. 100 beats/min.
   D. 120 beats/min.

257. Which location is recommended to assess the pulse of a 2-month-old child?

   A. Radial artery.
   B. Carotid artery.
   C. Apical impulse.
   D. Brachial artery.

258. What is the most common cause of cardiac arrest in children?

   A. Myocardial infarction.
   B. Trauma to the chest.
   C. Electrocution.
   D. Respiratory failure.

259. Which drugs may be administered via the endotracheal tube in the pediatric patient?

   A. Atropine, epinephrine, lidocaine.
   B. Atropine, sodium bicarbonate, epinephrine.
   C. Atropine, epinephrine.
   D. Atropine, epinephrine, calcium.

260. You are called to see a 1-month-old male infant with a two-day history of vomiting and diarrhea. Which of the following findings would be of the most concern?

   A. Respiratory rate of 56/min.
   B. Pulse rate of 150/min.
   C. Mottling of the extremities on crying.
   D. Sunken fontanelle.

Answers with Rationale

1. (D) Chronic bronchitis causes mucus plugs in the bronchioles leading to atelectasis and hypercarbia. Of all patients with COPD, those with chronic bronchitis are the most apt to function on hypoxic drive and are classically known as "blue bloaters" from being overweight and having a chronic cyanotic complexion.

2. (C) Emphysema destroys the alveolar walls resulting in a decrease in the number of alveoli and alveolar capillaries. The disease process breaks down the walls between alveoli, causing larger emphysema blebs, which are inelastic. This produces less surface area to exchange oxygen and leads to gradual intolerance for exercise. This patient is classically referred to as a "pink puffer," since the skin color is usually pink. The patient is also often thin with a barrel chest. (Note: Most COPD patients have both emphysema and chronic bronchitis, and it is rare to find an individual who has purely one or the other.)

3. (A) The goal for COPD patients in acute failure is to correct hypoxia, even though this may eliminate the hypoxic drive. Be prepared to intubate and ventilate the patient if this happens. Therapy may also include albuterol to improve bronchial air flow and alveolar ventilation, but the primary concern is the airway and oxygenation. Epinephrine is contraindicated.

4. (D) When COPD patients develop an infection, they produce more mucus than the normal individual. Since their respiratory status is usually marginal at best, this causes increased mucus plugging and atelectasis, resulting in hypoxia. These patients are also prone to spontaneously rupturing emphysema blebs causing pneumothorax, but this is less frequent. Pulmonary edema may cause respiratory failure, but it is usually due to left heart failure and not to the COPD.

5. (C) In the normal individual, respirations are stimulated by a rise in $PaCO_2$. Patients with chronic bronchitis are chronic CO_2 retainers. Therefore, elevated CO_2 levels cease to regulate respirations. The individuals depend on changes in PaO_2 to regulate respirations. This is known as the hypoxic drive. Hyperventilation, asthma, and carbon monoxide poisoning do not cause CO_2 retention.

6. (A) Due to chronic dyspnea, COPD patients use as many of their muscles as possible to get more air. This results in prominent accessory muscles and a barrel chest. Also, due to destruction of pulmonary capillary beds, blood backs up to the right heart, resulting in right heart failure. The output of the left heart is usually unaffected; therefore, left heart failure is uncommon.

7. (B) A positive history of heavy smoking, barrel chest, and/or use of accessory muscles should make you suspicious of COPD. While abnormal breath sounds, skin color, and nail beds may be present with COPD, they are nonspecific and may be indicative of other pathology. Left heart failure is not a result of COPD.

8. (A) The symptoms noted are classic signs of increased $PaCO_2$. The acutely hypoxic patient may present as agitated, combative, and disoriented. Symptoms of hypertension may include headache, GI disturbances, and drowsiness in addition to an elevated blood pressure.

9. (A) While all of these conditions may cause hypoxia, only a massive embolism commonly causes hypotension. The emboli lodge in a pulmonary artery and obstruct flow from the right heart to the lung and left heart.

10. (D) Pulmonary embolism can significantly reduce or halt blood flow through a pulmonary vessel. Consequently, blood is prevented from reaching the alveolar/capillary membranes where gas exchange can occur, resulting in a ventilation/perfusion mismatch (V/Q). The left ventricle does not fail; it is just receiving an inadequate amount of blood to pump.

11. (C) Classically in pulmonary embolism, a clot is dislodged from a deep vein in a lower extremity, then migrates to the right heart and into the pulmonary circulation. Arterial emboli may remain localized or may move to other organs, such as the brain or viscera. Pulmonary arteries return blood to the left heart.

12. (D) Asthma causes bronchospasm, which narrows bronchioles and decreases laminar air flow. It is also complicated by thick secretions. The alveoli of the asthmatic are intact. The patient usually does not retain CO_2, and generally moves air well until an attack of acute bronchospasm.

13. (A) When repeated doses of subcutaneous epinephrine do not relieve bronchospasm, this situation is referred to as status asthmaticus.

14. (D) The primary goal of management for the asthmatic patient is to relieve bronchospasm. This will improve alveolar ventilation. ECG monitoring, an intravenous line, and rehydration are secondary considerations.

15. (B) Steam conducts heat well and may cause burns to the lung mucosa. Since dry air is a poor conductor of heat, superheated dry air rarely causes burns of the lower airway by itself. Phosgene gas and carbon monoxide are both highly toxic, but do not produce thermal burns.

16. (A) Due to this patient's age and cardiac history, epinephrine is contraindicated. While her peak expiratory flow is unknown, she is able to talk without difficulty, which indicates she is moving air well. The most appropriate care is hydration, oxygenation, and careful monitoring during transportation.

17. (B) The standard dosage of epinephrine for bronchospasm is 0.3–0.5 mg of 1:1000 solution subcutaneously.

18. (C) Albuterol has gained increasing popularity as a first line therapy for the acute asthma attack. Nebulized therapy has proven generally more effective than parenteral therapy. Albuterol produces few cardiac side effects and is safe for frequent application. The availability of safe nebulized therapy has greatly reduced the use of aminophylline in the field with its potential side effects. Epinephrine may be considered subcutaneously, rather than intravenously. Steroids, such as methylprednisolone, have a delayed onset of action, and are not the first drug of choice.

19. (B) While each EMS system has a different approach to drug therapy, aminophylline in a dose of 250–500 mg over 20 minutes is generally considered safe. Consult with your Medical Control for local protocol.

20. (B) Due to the patient's history of fever, chills, productive cough, and lung consolidation, the paramedic should suspect a right lung pneumonia, which should be treated by oxygen, a KVO IV, monitoring, and transport. Use of Lasix would dehydrate this patient and worsen the lung consolidation. Morphine would depress the patient's respiratory

drive. Since the pain is pleuritic in nature and the history does not point to AMI, nitroglycerine is not indicated; and, since there are no arrhythmias, lidocaine is unnecessary. There is no acute bronchospasm; therefore, epinephrine and aminophylline are also not indicated.

21. (B) Pulse oximetry is a rapid measurement of oxygen saturation. The sensing unit is placed on the finger and transmits light through the vascular bed, determining the oxygen saturation of red blood cells. The pulse rate can also be monitored. PaO_2, hypercarbia, and hypocarbia are all measured by arterial blood gases.

22. (B) When more than one rib is fractured in more than one place, it results in an unstable segment of ribs that moves "paradoxically" with each breath and is known as flail chest. It may cause pneumothorax, pulmonary contusion, and decreased tidal volume, all leading to hypoxia.

23. (B) This patient presents a clinical picture of a left tension pneumothorax. Jugular venous distention is due to the high thoracic pressure inhibiting venous return. Air outside the lung builds in pressure, causing a mediastinal shift. The trachea has, therefore, shifted toward the right. Tracheal deviation is a late sign and is often not seen. Appropriate care would include oxygenation, control of the airway by endotracheal intubation, and needle thoracostomy (on the left) to relieve the tension pneumothorax. Pericardiocentesis is not indicated because you suspect tension pneumothorax, not a pericardial tamponade. Hyperventilation by bag-valve-mask device would increase the tension pneumothorax.

24. (B) Atelectasis refers to a collapse of alveoli, which are the main units of gas exchange. Collapsed, noninflated alveoli cannot exchange O_2/CO_2. Cardiac output decrease and dead space increase are not factors in hypoxia caused by atelectasis.

25. (A) Because rib fractures are so painful, patients do not breathe deeply enough. The drop in tidal volume causes nonventilated alveoli to collapse. Bronchospasm and bronchitis are not caused by rib fractures. Normal mucus production continues.

26. (B) A history of paresthesia in the hands, face, and feet and your physical findings of tachypnea and carpopedal spasm suggest respiratory alkalosis. The cause of the flexion in the hands and feet is carpopedal

spasm, not a seizure. *Caution*: Tachypnea, paresthesia, and anxiety are not exclusively due to hyperventilation. Be sure to consider other causes before using a rebreather bag. When in doubt, use oxygen.

27. (C) The diaphragm, which is the main muscle of breathing, separates the abdominal and thoracic cavities.

28. (C) The right lung has three lobes; the left has two.

29. (B) The normal partial pressures of O_2 and CO_2 in arterial blood are O_2 80–100 torr (mm Hg) and CO_2 35–45 torr.

30. (D) Hypoxia exists when the arterial oxygen tension is less than 60 torr. When the PaO_2 is greater than 60 torr, CO_2 becomes the primary stimulus for breathing. Normally hemoglobin is almost fully saturated with O_2. With a drop in PaO_2 to 50–60 torr, small decreases in PaO_2 result in substantial decreases in hemoglobin O_2 saturation.

31. (B) Small increases in $PaCO_2$ (1–2 torr) will cause an increase in the respiratory rate.

32. (A) The amount of physiologic "dead space" in the average adult male is 150 ml. This is important when ventilating apneic patients. Not all of the oxygen delivered is available for alveolar gas exchange. For emergency ventilation, a tidal volume of 10–15 cc/kg is necessary for adequate alveolar exchange and to compensate for "dead space."

33. (A) The primary center for respiratory control is in the medulla, which closely monitors CO_2 and pH. The aortic arch and other sites for chemoreceptors are most sensitive to oxygen. The cerebral cortex and cerebellum do not play a role in respiratory regulation.

34. (C) The normal pH for arterial blood is 7.40, with a range from 7.35 to 7.45.

35. (C) The peripheral chemoreceptors in the carotid body respond quickly to decreases in PaO_2 levels. They also respond to some extent to alterations in $PaCO_2$ and hydrogen ion concentrations.

36. (B) Tidal volume, or air exchange with each resting breath, is about 500 ml in the average person.

37. (D) Minute volume is determined by multiplying the tidal volume by the respiratory rate. With a tidal volume of 1100 ml and a respiratory rate of 20, the minute volume would be 22,000 ml.

38. (D) The first step in assessment of the chest is inspection. Inspection should include the degree of distress, posture or position of the patient, breathing pattern, and ability to speak. Establishing the general condition will allow the paramedic to optimally apply other assessment/management skills.

39. (A) Cheyne-Stokes breathing is the classic waxing and waning of respirations with short periods of apnea between. Neurologic hyperventilation is rapid but constant, without periods of apnea. Kussmaul's respirations are rapid and deep. Eupnea is normal breathing.

40. (D) This respiratory pattern is rapid and deep, characteristic of Kussmaul's respiration. This pattern usually indicates acidosis, and the patient is trying to eliminate CO_2. A conscious patient might feel dyspneic, but dyspnea is subjective information and would not be considered an objective finding of a respiratory pattern. Eupnea is normal breathing. Biot's respirations are characterized by agonal, gasping breaths, irregular in rate and depth.

41. (C) Breathing deeply with the mouth open increases laminar air flow and the intensity of breath sounds. During nose breathing, air becomes quite turbulent and this softens sounds considerably. Normal tidal volumes are acceptable, but deep breathing improves assessment.

42. (B) While rapid respiratory assessment usually includes a quick check of the posterior bases, complete respiratory assessment always includes listening to each apex and base, anterior and posterior. If the patient cannot sit up or roll over, listen to the anterior and lateral chest.

43. (C) Since lung tissue containing alveoli and terminal bronchioles cover most of the pleural surface, vesicular sounds are generally auscultated. Bronchial sounds are heard over the trachea, and broncho-vesicular are heard over the bronchi along the sternum.

44. (C) Stridor, a high-pitched crowing sound, is caused by upper airway obstruction. Laryngeal edema and croup are accompanied by stridor.

45. (A) In addition to being described as "fine, moist sounds," rales are also described as having the quality of crackling or bubbling, "sand dropping on a tin can," or "hair rubbed by one's ear." Usually, rales are caused by air rushing into alveoli/terminal bronchioles that are filled with fluid or are atelectatic and are "popping" open. The rales of pulmonary edema are usually heard first at the bases of the lungs posteriorly. Rhonchi are usually caused by fluid or mucus that is partially obstructing the bronchi or the throat and are rumbling or rattling in quality. Whistling, high-pitched sounds that are heard primarily on expiration are called wheezes. Wheezing is due to air rushing through bronchioles that are constricted by edema or foreign materials, through a bronchus obstructed by a foreign object, or through bronchi that are in spasm, as in asthma.

46. (B) Irritation of the pleura commonly results in sharp chest pain, which varies with depth of inspiration. Pneumothorax, pulmonary embolism, and pleurisy often present with this type of pain. Acute bronchospasm usually results in a feeling of tightness in the chest and shortness of breath. The pain of AMI is classically described as a pressure in the chest that may radiate to the arms, neck, jaw, etc. and is not usually associated with dyspnea, unless acute left heart failure or pulmonary edema is present. Bronchial obstruction results in dyspnea and use of accessory muscles to aid breathing.

47. (D) Feeling of shortness of breath is a subjective feeling that the patient experiences. It may or may not be accompanied by tachypnea. Frightened appearance, flaring of the nostrils (nares), and intercostal muscle retraction are all objective physical signs of respiratory distress.

48. (A) The healthy respiratory center exerts a fine control on $PaCO_2$ levels to maintain an arterial level of 40 mm Hg. An increased $PaCO_2$ level stimulates the medulla and peripheral chemoreceptors to increase the rate and depth of respirations to facilitate carbon dioxide elimination.

49. (B) The smallest functional unit of the respiratory system is the alveolus. Capillaries surround the alveoli and make gas exchange possible through a process of diffusion. The bifurcation of the trachea into the right and left mainstem bronchi is termed the carina. Between the lateral and median glossoepiglottic folds, in the hypopharynx, is a depression referred to as the vallecula epiglottica. The bronchioles are the

smallest divisions of the bronchi, which divide further into the alveolar ducts within the lungs.

50. (D) Central neurogenic hyperventilation is caused by injury to the lower portions of the brain stem and is a late sign of brain herniation syndrome. Cheyne-Stokes respirations is a periodic increase and decrease in respiratory volume separated by periods of apnea. Kussmaul's respiration, where breathing is increased in depth and rate, is the result of diabetic ketoacidosis. Eupneic ventilation is a normal respiratory pattern.

51. (A) Stridor or a "crowing" sound on inspiration is generally associated with upper airway obstruction due to epiglottitis, croup, laryngeal edema, injuries, or anaphylaxis. Lower airway obstructions such as asthma, bronchiolitis, and pneumonia commonly cause prolonged exhalation, wheezing, dyspnea, nasal flaring, and retractions of the chest wall.

52. (A) Atmospheric gases contain 21% oxygen, 78% nitrogen, 0.04% carbon dioxide, and 0.50% water.

53. (C) According to AHA guidelines, six to ten abdominal thrusts should be delivered in rapid succession. Repeated abdominal thrusts may be more successful than single, well-spaced attempts delivered slowly. Repeated attempts may increase the pressure behind the foreign body and dislodge it. If unsuccessful, check for foreign body, attempt to ventilate, and repeat the sequence. Visualize the airway with a laryngoscope and remove any visible foreign body with McGill forceps.

54. (D) Signs and symptoms of carbon monoxide poisoning include headaches, irritability, errors in judgment, vomiting, chest pain, confusion, agitation, loss of coordination, loss of consciousness, and seizures. Children may have an increased susceptibility to carbon monoxide poisoning. Given the lack of apparent history for other causes of seizure, this particular setting, and the symptoms exhibited by the parents, suspect carbon monoxide poisoning.

55. (D) The aortic and pulmonic, semilunar valves, are open during ventricular systole (contraction). The atrioventricular valves, mitral and tricuspid, are open during ventricular diastole (filling), which allows the blood to flow from the atria into the ventricles.

56. (B) The endocardium forms the inner surface of the heart. The myocardium, or middle layer of the heart wall, is the muscle responsible for heart contraction. The pericardium is the sac that encloses the heart. The epicardium is the outer layer of the heart and is the same as the visceral pericardium.

57. (C) The chordae tendinae extend to the papillary muscles along the ventricular wall, and support the valves during ventricular contraction to prevent backflow of blood into the atrium. The semilunar valves prevent backflow from the aorta or pulmonary artery into the ventricles during ventricular relaxation. The sinuses of Valsalva protect the coronary orifices from occlusion by the valve leaflets when the aortic valve opens.

58. (C) With reference to the coats of arteries, the outer coat is called tunica adventitia; the middle coat is tunica media; and the inner coat is tunica intima. Atherosclerosis is a progressive disease which involves the tunica intima. Deposition of fats (lipids) and cholesterol stimulates an injury response in the vessel wall and damage to the tunica media occurs. Calcium is subsequently deposited with resultant plaque formation. Small hemorrhages into the plaque may occur and are followed by more scarring and fibrosis.

59. (A) Cardiac output is the amount of blood pumped by the heart each minute. Cardiac output is dependent upon the relationship between two variables: heart rate and stroke volume. Stroke volume is the amount of blood pumped out of the heart during each cardiac cycle. Cardiac output can be computed by multiplying the stroke volume by the heart rate per minute (cardiac output = stroke volume X heart rate per minute). Preload is the fiber stretch at the end of diastole. Afterload refers to the degree of myocardial fiber stretch during systole.

60. (A) Immediately following myocardial depolarization, there is a brief interval known as the absolute refractory period, during which the heart muscle is incapable of responding to any stimulus. A relative refractory period follows, during which the myocardium will respond only to strong stimulation. The Frank-Starling mechanism refers to the fact that when the myocardium is stretched, it contracts more forcefully and becomes more efficient as a pump. There is no electromechanical threshold. (A threshold is the point at which a stimulus will cause a cell to respond.)

61. (B) The cholinergic response is produced by parasympathetic stimulation. Stimulation of parasympathetic fibers causes the release of acetylcholine. Acetylcholine mediates the transmission of the neural impulse to the cardiac receptors and triggers a cholinergic or vagal response. The adrenergic response involves an acceleration of the heart rate, increased speed of impulse transmission through the node, and increased force of myocardial contraction. Anticholinergic response is the blocking of impulses that travel through the parasympathetic nerves. Alpha-receptors are found in all blood vessels except capillaries, and vasoconstriction occurs when these receptors are stimulated.

62. (D) The SA node is normally the physiological pacemaker because it has the fastest rate of impulse formation (60–100/min). Impulses are conducted by the internodal pathways to the AV node (or junctional tissue). After a slight delay to maximally fill the ventricles, impulses are conducted through the AV bundle (or Bundle of His). Depolarizing both ventricles is accomplished by conduction through right and left bundle branches to the most rapid conducting tissue, the Purkinje system.

63. (A) Closure of the tricuspid valve prevents backflow of blood to the right atrium. The valves controlling the flow of blood from the atria to the ventricles are the tricuspid and mitral valves. The three leaflets of the tricuspid valve are forced shut by the increased pressure and kept closed during the ventricular contraction to prevent backflow of blood into the right atrium. The mitral valve consists of two leaflets, or cusps, and serves the same function for the left atrium and ventricle.

64. (A) As the wave of electrical activity spreads throughout the atria, depolarization occurs. This is identified on the ECG as a P-wave. After a brief delay in the AV node, depolarization of the ventricles occurs, resulting in a QRS complex. Ventricular recovery, or repolarization, begins with the S-T segment and is complete with the end of the T-wave.

65. (C) Collateral circulation refers to the gradual formation of interconnections between the coronary arteries to supply additional blood. Coronary circulation comprises the three major vessels supplying blood to the myocardium. Extracorporeal circulation is circulation of blood through an external device such as an artificial kidney machine or heart lung machine. The lymphatic system consists of the lymph capillaries, lymphatic vessels, lymphatic ducts, and lymph nodes.

66. (C) The left main coronary artery has two major branches: anterior descending and circumflex arteries. The circumflex artery supplies circulation to the left atrium and ventricle. Posterior descending and marginal branch are the two major divisions of the right main coronary artery. The right main coronary artery supplies the right atrium and ventricle.

67. (A) Automaticity is a property of the heart muscle tissue (in specific pacemaker cells) that allows it to generate its own electrical impulse without stimulation from nerves. Contractility refers to the ability of a muscle fiber to contract independently in response to a stimulus. Conductivity is the ability to transmit an impulse that has been initiated and passed along cell membranes. The conductivity of cardiac muscle fiber provides for smooth and efficient contraction of the heart's muscle mass. Excitability is the ability to respond to a stimulus and initiate an impulse.

68. (B) Norepinephrine is a potent peripheral vasoconstrictor (Alpha adrenergic). Sympatholytic agents block receptor sites. Alpha blockade would result in vasodilation.

69. (B) Pharmacological therapy is indicated only when the bradycardia results in adverse alterations of hemodynamic stability. Well-conditioned athletes frequently have very slow pulse rates. Signs and/or symptoms indicating a need to treat this dysrhythmia include: (1) hypotension (BP <90); (2) congestive heart failure; (3) ventricular escape beats; (4) chest pain; (5) dyspnea; or (6) altered level of consciousness. In the event that treatment is necessary, atropine sulfate 0.5 mg IV push every 5 minutes up to a maximum of 2.0 mg is the initial management.

70. (D) Usually 0.5 to 1.0 mg of a 1:10,000 solution of epinephrine is administered intravenously in resuscitation efforts. When an endotracheal tube is in place, 1.0 mg of 1:10,000 solution may be instilled directly into the tracheobronchial tree. A larger dose of drug is needed to achieve pressor responses when endotracheal instillation is used. The subcutaneous route is not utilized during cardiac arrest.

71. (D) A normal sinus rhythm is indicated by a regular rhythm. Each QRS complex is preceded by a normal P-wave; the P-R interval is 0.12 to 0.20

sec and regular; the QRS duration is 0.10 sec or less. In first-degree AV block, the P-R interval is prolonged beyond 0.20 sec; in Mobitz I or Wenckebach, the P-R interval lengthens progressively until a QRS complex is dropped. Sinus arrhythmia is an irregular rhythm.

72. (A) The patient is in electromechanical dissociation (EMD), which is defined as organized electrical activity on the ECG without a palpable pulse. Hypovolemia is a potential cause that may be assessed through the administration of a fluid challenge. During the first ten minutes of resuscitation, the trachea has been intubated, an IV line established, and epinephrine administered. Although sodium bicarbonate therapy is considered at this time, without an estimated weight or arterial blood gas reports, 100 mEq could be an excessive dose. The route of epinephrine administration is probably not related to the lack of desired effect. In the presence of a bradyrhythmia that does not respond to initial therapy, atropine may be considered appropriate to increase the heart rate. Other potential causes of EMD include cardiac tamponade, tension pneumothorax, hypoxemia, acidosis, and pulmonary embolism.

73. (B) The SA node is the physiological pacemaker of the heart because it has the most rapid inherent firing rate at 60–100 beats per minute. The atrioventricular node inherent rate is 40–60 per minute. The slowest inherent rate is in the Purkinje system with a rate of 20–40 beats per minute. Under normal circumstances, depolarization should result in myocardial contraction. However, myocardial damage (e.g., infarction) may prevent the normal response, resulting in EMD, or electromechanical dissociation. The cardiac cycle consists normally of systole (0.28 seconds) and diastole (0.52 seconds), which require a total of 0.80 seconds.

74. (D) Angina and infarction may produce the same complaint of pain; however, the elevation of the ST segment on the electrocardiogram indicates the presence of myocardial injury consistent with an acute myocardial infarction. Although heat exhaustion may exacerbate symptoms in a patient with coronary artery disease, it does not produce waveform changes on the electrocardiogram. Dull pain is not characteristic of a dissecting aneurysm; the pain is described as tearing or ripping. Unlike infarction pain, dissections produce pain that is most intense at its onset.

75. (A) Due to the vasodilating effects exerted by this drug, sublingual nitroglycerin should not be utilized in the presence of hypotension. A na-

sal cannula is generally well tolerated and, with an oxygen flow of 6 liters per minute, delivers a concentration of 25–40%. Ventricular fibrillation is the leading cause of sudden cardiac death for the patient experiencing an acute myocardial infarction. Because this lethal dysrhythmia may develop without warning ectopy, prophylactic therapy with lidocaine should be initiated with an initial bolus of 1.5 mg/kg followed by an infusion of 2–4 mg/min. Due to the high occurrence of ventricular fibrillation and other serious dysrhythmias during the early hours of infarction, continuous monitoring of the electrocardiogram is essential.

76. (B) A relationship between body size and the energy needed for defibrillation has been shown between pediatric and adult patients. It is clear that infants and small children require less energy than adults. However, the range of adult size and weight has not been demonstrated to be clinically important in determining the energy level required for defibrillation.

77. (B) Paddle electrode placement is critical for successful defibrillation. One electrode is placed just to the right of the upper sternum and below the clavicle. The other is positioned lateral to the left nipple with the center of the electrode in the left midaxillary line. This placement maximizes the flow of the electrical current through the myocardium.

78. (D) Atrial fibrillation results from a rapid, chaotic electrical impulse formation disorder within the atrium. Due to the absence of organized atrial impulse formation and the rapid rate at which impulses are generated, the ventricular rhythm is always irregular (irregular RRI). The electrical disorder also results in the replacement of P-waves by F-waves which occur at a rate of ≥350 per minute. Sinus tachycardia requires the presence of identifiable P-waves, 1:1 P:QRS ratio, constant PRI >0.11 sec, and uniform P-wave shape consistent with the monitoring lead. Atrial flutter is characterized by the presence of F-waves. When the atrial rate of impulse formation is 250–350 per minute, P-waves lose their characteristic rounded shape and become saw-toothed in appearance At this point, they are referred to as F-waves. There is insufficient evidence on the ECG tracing to identify a second-degree AV block Type I.

79. (A) The presenting signs and symptoms and the atrial fibrillation in this situation are characteristic of congestive heart failure (CHF). Although classified as an analgesic, morphine sulfate is beneficial in the treatment

of acute pulmonary edema because it increases venous capacitance which decreases venous return (preload) to the failing heart. A mild degree of arterial vasodilation is another beneficial action of morphine sulfate in this situation. Morphine creates a physiological rotating tourniquet effect by reducing the preload. Diazepam (Valium) exerts no beneficial actions in pulmonary edema. Verapamil is a calcium channel blocker. It reduces the blood pressure and may worsen CHF in patients with left ventricular dysfunction. Propranolol (Inderal) is a Beta-adrenergic blocker and may also exacerbate CHF.

80. (D) Oxygen is the first drug of choice when treating ventricular ectopy because hypoxemia is a major contributing factor to myocardial irritability. If there is no response to the oxygen, lidocaine therapy should be instituted. Atropine is not indicated in this situation since the ectopy is not compensating for a bradycardia. Although pain causes a sympathetic response which could potentially result in ventricular ectopy, the administration of morphine sulfate will not improve oxygenation of the myocardium and should not be considered as first-line drug therapy.

81. (A) Bretylium tosylate is recommended when (1) lidocaine and defibrillation fail to convert ventricular fibrillation, (2) ventricular fibrillation recurs despite lidocaine, as in this case, or (3) lidocaine and procainamide have failed to control ventricular tachycardia associated with a pulse. The initial dosage is 5 mg/kg circulated for 2 minutes with CPR, followed by electrical defibrillation. If ventricular fibrillation continues, Bretylium may be repeated at 10 mg/kg every 15–30 minutes for a maximum dose of 30 mg/kg. Propranolol is indicated in certain situations when ventricular dysrhythmias are due to excessive Beta stimulation. It is not recommended when cardiac function is severely depressed, as in the case of cardiac arrest.

82. (C) When sodium bicarbonate is used without the benefit of arterial blood gas reports, the initial dose should be 1 mEq/kg followed by 0.5 mEq/kg every 10 minutes thereafter.

83. (C) The prehospital drug of choice for managing cardiogenic shock is dopamine. The initial rate of a dopamine infusion in this situation is 5 mcg/kg due to profound hypotension. The patient's weight in kilograms (165 divided by 2.2) is 75 kg. The total dose per minute is 75 kg multiplied by 5 mcg/kg/min or 375 mcg/min. Mixing 800 mg (or

800,000 micrograms, mcg) into 500 ml of solution yields a concentration of 1600 mcg per ml. Microdrop tubing delivers 60 gtts/ml. Therefore, 60 gtts = 1600 mg. Use the following formula:

$$\frac{\text{Desired Dose}}{\text{Dose on Hand}} \times \text{Vehicle} = \text{Volume Administered}$$

The solution is:

$$\frac{375 \text{ mcg/min}}{1600 \text{ mcg/ml}} \times \frac{60 \text{ gtts/ml}}{1} = \frac{22{,}500 \text{ gtts/min}}{1600} = 14 \text{ gtts/min}$$

Dobutamine is administered at 2.5–20 mcg/kg/min. Norepinephrine, when indicated, is started at 2 mcg/min. The usual adult range is 2–12 mcg/min, although higher doses may be required to maintain an adequate blood pressure. Prophylactic lidocaine is given at 1.5 mg/kg bolus followed by a continuous infusion of 2–4 mg/min. However, this patient's hypoperfusion status would require a reduced dose to prevent toxicity.

84. (C) Morphine is the analgesic of choice for the pain associated with an acute myocardial infarction (AMI). It should be administered in small incremental doses (2 to 5 mg) as often as every 5 minutes until the desired response is achieved. Titrating the dosage in this manner reduces the possibility of respiratory depression and hypotension. Whereas Tridil (intravenous nitroglycerin) and sublingual nitroglycerin are used in the management of chest pain associated with AMI, they are not classified as analgesics. Nitrites and nitrates relax the vascular smooth muscle. Amrinone (Inocor Lactate Injection) produces effects similar to dobutamine. Amrinone is a nonadrenergic cardiotonic agent, not an analgesic.

85. (B) The initial dose of furosemide is 0.5 to 1.0 mg/kg slow IV push. The patient's weight in kilograms (121 divided by 2.2) is 55 kg. The dose range is 55 kg multiplied by 0.5 mg/kg = 27.5 mg and 55 kg multiplied by 1.0 mg/kg = 55 mg.

86. (D) Firm paddle-to-skin contact pressure has the potential to decrease transthoracic resistance, a factor contributing to the success of defibrillation attempts. Therefore, apply firm pressure of 25 pounds to the paddles when the countershock is delivered. It is important that the operator exert a downward pressure with a squeezing action rather

than leaning on the paddles. Leaning may result in the paddles sliding off the chest.

87. (C) Prior to defibrillating ventricular fibrillation a second time, you must make certain that the patient does not have a pulse. Poor paddle-to-skin contact during a quick-look may produce artifact that mimics ventricular fibrillation. Once it has been verified that the patient remains pulseless, the paddles are recharged and defibrillation is repeated at 360 joules. If there is no response, pharmacological therapy is instituted and ECG monitoring electrodes are put in place.

88. (D) Calcium administration is contraindicated for digitalis toxicity because it potentiates the effect of digitalis and contributes to the development of dysrhythmias. Hyperkalemia often results from acute metabolic and respiratory acidosis due to an extracellular shift of potassium. Calcium quickly counteracts the neuromuscular effects of hyperkalemia. Multiple blood transfusions are one of many causes of hypocalcemia. Citrate (which is added to the donor blood to prevent coagulation) bonds with the recipient's serum calcium and prevents its utilization. In the presence of calcium channel blocker toxicity (Verapamil), the administration of calcium chloride increases the calcium ion passage across the slow, or calcium, channel.

89. (B) Since the ground or reference electrode does not provide cardiac information for use in the actual recording, it may be placed anywhere on the body.

90. (B) The ventricular ectopy present in this tracing is compensatory and not competitive activity. Ventricular escape beats are associated with a profound bradycardia. This situation requires the administration of atropine sulfate to increase the heart rate rather than acute suppressive therapy with lidocaine hydrochloride. The objective of the therapy is to treat the cause of the ectopy, which is a bradycardia.

91. (A) Torsade de pointes (twisting of the points) is a specific type of ventricular tachycardia characterized by the changing polarity of ventricular complexes (Q-S complex → QRS complex → Q-S complex, etc.). Three or more consecutive premature ventricular contractions with a rate greater than 100/min defines ventricular tachycardia. Since there are no apparent P-waves or indications of hidden Ps on Ts, this rhythm

is determined to be ventricular in origin. Ventricular fibrillation is chaotic and lacks the organized complexes demonstrated in this ECG.

92. (A) The ECG tracing reveals an electronic ventricular pacemaker rhythm with a 1:1 pacemaker spike to QRS response. Increased duration of the QRS complex is due to the placement of the pacemaker electrode (apex of the right ventricle). This dysrhythmia requires no prehospital intervention.

93. (A) The inability to ascertain a blood pressure and the pulse deficit indicate this patient is hemodynamically unstable secondary to the supraventricular tachycardia. This necessitates the need for electrical management. Vagal maneuvers, followed by Verapamil and subsequent Beta blocker therapy, are indicated for supraventricular tachycardia when the patient is not exhibiting signs or symptoms of perfusion deficit.

94. (A) Since the premature ventricular ectopy responded to the lidocaine bolus, a lidocaine infusion must be initiated to maintain a therapeutic blood level of the medication. The maximum bolus dose is 3 mg/kg which requires a maintenance infusion of 4 mg/min. Some prehospital protocols utilize a rebolus regime. If the ectopy had not responded to lidocaine, procainamide and bretylium would have been used respectively. Atropine is administered for bradycardia.

95. (C) While atrial flutter is one example of supraventricular tachycardia, the characteristic jagged, saw-toothed flutter (F) waves are apparent on this tracing. Atrial flutter may result in a regular or irregular ventricular rhythm. The irregularity of the R-R intervals is caused by the variable conduction through the AV node.

96. (D) Dopamine, norepinephrine, and epinephrine are naturally occurring catecholamines and possess both Alpha and Beta stimulating properties. The Alpha receptors are located predominantly in the vasculature and, when stimulated, result in vasoconstriction. $Beta_1$ receptors are located predominantly in the myocardium. Stimulation of these receptors produces positive inotropic, chronotropic, and dromotropic effects. $Beta_1$ receptor sites are located in the smooth muscle, including the vasculature. These tissues respond to $Beta_2$ activity with relaxation (e.g., bronchodilatation and vasodilation).

97. (A) Nitronox is a blended mixture of 50% nitrous oxide and 50% oxygen. When inhaled, it has potent analgesic properties which quickly dissipate within 2–5 minutes after discontinuation. Since it is self-administered, maximal dose is achieved when the patient drops the hand-held delivery mask. Nausea and vomiting may occur in susceptible individuals but are untoward, not therapeutic, effects.

98. (D) Normally the time of ventricular filling (diastole) is approximately twice that of ejection (systole). In the presence of tachycardia, diastolic times are greatly reduced. This results in inadequate ventricular filling which reduces the stroke volume (the amount of blood ejected with each contraction) as well as the cardiac output (stroke volume X pulse rate). Ultimately the blood pressure is reduced since the blood pressure is determined by the cardiac output multiplied by the peripheral vascular resistance. If there is insufficient blood in the ventricle at the time of systole, the pulse will not be palpable. The discrepancy between the ECG rate and the palpated pulse is referred to as the pulse deficit.

99. (C) The waveform abnormality in this ECG is the high, tent-like T-wave. (T-waves should not exceed 5 mm in any of the leads.) Hyperkalemia (excessive serum potassium level) increases the height of the T-wave. Hypokalemia (deficient serum potassium level) results in the appearance of prominent U-waves on the ECG. Whereas potassium is responsible for the resting membrane potential of the heart, sodium is responsible for the action potential. Hyponatremia and hypernatremia are deficient and excessive sodium levels.

100. (A) The presence of acute right heart failure (indicated by jugular vein distention, or JVD) and pleuritic chest pain (aggravated by respirations) together with the recent surgical history are highly indicative of pulmonary embolism. If the embolus is large enough to prevent cardiopulmonary circulation, cardiac arrest is inevitable. The pain associated with a dissecting aortic aneurysm is reported by the patient as a tearing or ripping pain that is generally not associated with respiratory effort. Although JVD is commonly seen in the presence of a tension pneumothorax, it is not a result of spontaneous pneumothorax.

101. (A) Since the patient has not been taking the Lasix (diuretic) but has continued to take the Slo-K (potassium supplement), he is a candidate for the hyperkalemia evidenced on the ECG (high, tent-like T-waves).

The balance between a therapeutic and toxic digitalis level (Lanoxin) and potassium is critical to maintaining a sinus rhythm. The premature atrial activity present on the ECG indicates the toxicity of the digitalis. Since the premature atrial contractions (PAC) occur after every sinus complex, this pattern would be referred to as bigeminal. Sinus arrhythmia is present when the sinus rate increases with inspiration and decreases with expiration. This is due to vagal stimulation and is frequently seen in the pediatric age group. The fibrillatory waves (f waves) which characterize atrial fibrillation are not present on the ECG. Wandering atrial pacemaker would be diagnosed by a changing in the P-wave configuration.

102. (B) The missing QRS complexes indicate second-degree heart block. Because there are two consecutive constant PR intervals prior to the dropped QRS with a QRS duration of greater than 0.11 seconds, this is a second-degree AV heart block Type II (or Mobitz II). Third-degree block is characterized by regular P-P intervals, regular R-R intervals, and variable PR intervals because there is no A-V relationship. Second-degree AV block Type I (or Mobitz I) presents with increasing PRI and decreasing R-R interval until the dropped beat. The pattern is then repeated. Although there is an increased PRI duration, first-degree AV block does not involve dropped QRS complexes.

103. (A) The ECG reveals an underlying sinus rhythm, with well-defined P-waves at regular intervals. The ectopic beats are greater than 0.12 seconds, are not preceded by P-waves, and therefore, are premature ventricular contractions.

104. (D) Adequate oxygenation of the myocardium can considerably reduce ischemia and pain. Ischemic tissue is also more prone to ectopy. High-concentration oxygen therapy may reduce chest pain and eliminate PVCs and is the initial treatment of choice in the suspected AMI. Oxygenation often obviates the need to administer other drugs. Because the patient is currently hypotensive, administration of additional nitroglycerin or morphine is not indicated. Administration of oxygen by cannula at 6 L/min will deliver an FiO_2 of only ±40%.

105. (C) Initially, the best approach is to avoid additional pharmacologic intervention until you have had an opportunity to observe the effects of placing the patient supine, allowing the nitroglycerin to wear off and the

oxygen to work. If hypotension or ectopy continues, additional interventions would be considered.

106. (D) Due to the onset of symptoms without provocation, the nature of the pain, and previous history, either unstable angina or AMI must be suspected. Initially, the hypotension would be presumed to be the result of the self-administration of nitroglycerin. Other causes must be investigated if the patient is still hypotensive after the peak action time of nitroglycerin has passed.

107. (B) The rhythm is a narrow complex tachycardia with a rate of 100–120/min, with well-defined P-waves, and it is regular. Therefore, it is sinus tachycardia.

108. (D) The most appropriate treatment is a fluid challenge and transportation to a hospital where prompt surgical intervention is available. The initial history suggests an aneurism with hypotension. Pain radiating to the back and disparity in radial pulses are classic findings. Syncope after standing suggests postural hypotension. The patient's pulse is 100 and is borderline tachycardia. The diastolic blood pressure is elevated, which is common in patients who are in compensated shock. The cardiac rate is not fast or slow enough to produce hypotension due to poor cardiac output.

109. (D) Hypovolemia due to occult bleeding should be suspected as the cause of the tachycardia. Stokes-Adams syndrome is syncope secondary to a rhythm that results in poor cardiac output, such as a bradycardia or supraventricular tachycardia. The patient's cardiac rate is not fast or slow enough to consider this as the cause of the hypotension.

110. (B) The initial approach to this patient is high-concentration oxygen. A nonrebreathing mask delivers high concentrations. A cannula is a low-to medium-concentration device. IV access should be established and an IV of D$_5$W started. D$_5$W is utilized because it does not stay in circulating volume.

111. (D) High-concentration oxygen frequently decreases or eliminates ischemic chest pain because of increased off-loading to the ischemic myocardium. Oxygen is the first management priority. If pain continues, nitroglycerin is indicated, then morphine.

112. (D) The underlying cardiac rate is less than 60/min and there are ectopic beats. The QRS measures are greater than 0.12 seconds and not preceded by P-waves. In addition, the QRS complexes are falling late in the cardiac cycle. Therefore, they are ventricular escape beats due to a slow ventricular rate.

113. (C) Although it is tempting to treat the ectopy with lidocaine, the correct approach is to increase the underlying cardiac rate with atropine. Once the rate increases, the ventricles will depolarize frequently enough to eliminate the escape mechanism. Isoproterenol is last resort for symptomatic bradycardias.

114. (A) The rate, P-R interval, and QRS width are all normal. The interpretation is normal sinus rhythm.

115. (D) She should be strongly encouraged to allow you to continue with your assessment and with transportation to the hospital. Syncope in an elderly patient is a "wolf in sheep's clothing"! It should always be handled as an ALS work-up with the physical assessment vectored to detect positive findings in the neurologic, cardiovascular, and musculoskeletal systems. Her specific history of "palpitations" for the last week should make one suspect episodes of paroxysmal supraventricular or ventricular tachycardia. It is not uncommon for patients on diuretic therapy to become hypokalemic and develop lethal dysrhythmias.

116. (A) Due to the history of recent palpitations, Stokes-Adams syndrome should be strongly suspected. Stokes-Adams syndrome is a condition caused by heart block and characterized by sudden attacks of unconsciousness. Bystander accounts do not suggest tonic-clonic movement, and there are no physical signs of seizure. The patient is neurologically intact and has no lingering evidence of brain ischemia. Wernicke-Korsakoff syndrome is mental deterioration secondary to thiamine depletion.

117. (C) While this patient does not exhibit a condition that requires aggressive intervention, she should be oxygenated and IV access established in the event that her condition deteriorates.

118. (B) The narrow complexes and rate of greater than 160/min indicate a supraventricular tachycardia (SVT). It cannot be called a paroxysmal

tachycardia because the strip does not demonstrate that the rhythm abruptly starts or terminates. Since the complexes are narrow, less than 0.12 seconds, they originate in the atria, not the ventricles.

119. (B) Since the patient is not hypotensive and there is no evidence of cardiac ischemia, his condition is considered to be "stable." However, he has significant symptoms, and his condition could deteriorate. An attempt should be made to terminate the dysrhythmia. Generally speaking, the treatment techniques progress in potential risk to the patient. Vagal maneuvers such as a Valsalva or carotid sinus massage (CSM) are the initial lines of treatment. If vagal maneuvers are unsuccessful, Verapamil is the treatment of choice. A newer drug, Adenosine, may be used. Adenosine is useful in patients with Wolf-Parkinson-White syndrome, and hypotension is not a side effect. The last treatment of choice is synchronized cardioversion after sedation with a benzodiazepine such as Versed or Valium.

120. (A) Prior to performing carotid sinus massage, the equality of carotid pulses must be palpated and the neck auscultated for bruits. Unequal carotid pulses indicate narrowing of the carotid arteries and contraindicate CSM. A carotid bruit (noise like a Korotkoff sound heard with each arterial pulsation) also indicates carotid narrowing. In either situation, CSM could break off a plaque, which might enter cerebral circulation and cause a stroke, or interrupt blood flow through the artery. Prior to using Verapamil, a history of Wolf-Parkinson-White syndrome must be determined.

121. (C) In some cases, the patient may convert to asystole or a very slow bradycardia. Successful vagal maneuvers cause parasympathetic stimulation that can result in gradual slowing of the rate. Whenever an attempt is made to terminate SVT, be prepared to resuscitate! Be prepared to ventilate, give atropine, and do CPR if necessary.

122. (C) The rhythm is atrial fibrillation. The rhythm is irregularly irregular, no P-waves are visible, and the baseline shows fibrillatory waves. There is organized ventricular activity, but no organized atrial activity. The rate is not fast enough for SVT. If this were a sinus rhythm with PACs, P-waves would be present and precede each QRS complex.

123. (B) This patient's pulse oximeter reading indicates a saturation of 91%; this indicates a PaO2 of slightly more than 60 torr. According to the oxy-

gen-hemoglobin dissociation curve, even when the PaO_2 is 60 torr, the hemoglobin is 90% saturated with oxygen. A patient is considered to be hypoxic when the PaO_2 is 60 torr or less. When assessing an oximeter, 90% saturation is a key level! *SpO_2 less than 90 means hypoxia.*

124. (C) High concentration oxygen via nonrebreathing mask is the initial treatment while getting the resuscitation equipment ready. This patient is in respiratory failure, as evidenced by the respiratory rate, restlessness, and SpO_2 of near 90%. However, since she can communicate verbally, she is moving some air. If she has an adequate minute volume, the oxygen can help significantly to improve the hypoxia, thus eliminating the need for ventilation/intubation. Look for signs of improvement such as decreasing restlessness and an improved SpO_2. If the patient's SpO_2 falls below 90 and she becomes more restless or obtunded, ventilation/intubation may become necessary. Oxygen by cannula and simple mask deliver only medium concentrations, not enough to rapidly correct hypoxia in a patient in respiratory failure.

125. (B) The patient presents a clinical picture of pulmonary edema, not infection or pneumonia. Therefore, the patient should be treated with furosemide. Morphine can be useful also, but it may depress respirations and should not be first-line treatment for the patient. Lidocaine can be given prophylactically, but it is not the initial priority because the patient does not exhibit ventricular ectopy. The patient does not have SVT requiring Verapamil.

126. (D) The interpretation is sinus bradycardia with first-degree AV block. The underlying rate is ±40/min and the P-R interval is greater than 0.20.

127. (B) The hypotension is probably causing some of the patient's symptoms. The initial presumption should be that the hypotension is due to poor cardiac output from the slow rate. Initial efforts must be made to increase the rate with atropine. Furosemide may be indicated later if the pressure improves and/or if the patient develops acute respiratory failure. Isoproterenol is second or third line therapy for bradycardia. Dopamine is indicated if hypotension persists after the rate exceeds 60–70/min. Cardiogenic shock would then be presumed to be the cause of the hypotension.

128. (D) The patient's rate has now increased to greater than 60/min, and the hypotension and symptoms persist. At this point, dopamine given

in the Beta ranges is indicated. Dopamine in low doses dilates the renal arteries. In medium doses it causes an increase in inotropic effect and is the desirable range for pump failure. The higher-dose ranges cause an Alpha effect and increase resistance and cardiac workload. When administering dopamine, observe the patient's skin and capillary beds to detect pallor—indication that the dopamine is causing vasoconstriction and an increase in afterload.

129. (B) The rate is over 100/min and less than 150/min. There are regular R-R and P-R intervals. The rhythm is sinus tachycardia.

130. (D) While both nifedipine and Verapamil are calcium blockers, nifedipine is the drug of choice for hypertensive crisis. Both furosemide and nitroglycerin can be used to transiently decrease blood pressure in a patient in hypertensive crisis.

131. (C) The P-R intervals are progressively longer until one of the P-waves is not conducted to the atria and is dropped. The R-R interval is progressively longer and is irregular. The rhythm is a second-degree Mobitz I, or Wenckebach.

132. (C) The second-degree Mobitz I is more likely to respond to atropine than is a Mobitz II, a higher grade block that can progress to complete heart block. Transthoracic pacing and isoproterenol are second or third line treatments for symptomatic bradycardias and blocks. Since hypovolemia is not suspected as the underlying cause of the hypotension, a fluid challenge is not appropriate.

133. (D) Glucagon is a naturally occurring hormone secreted by the alpha cells in the pancreatic islets of Langerhans and is available as a parenteral medication. It is referred to as an endogenous hyperglycemic factor because its actions are responsible for increasing the serum glucose level. This is accomplished primarily by stimulating breakdown of liver glycogen into glucose. This process is referred to as glycogenolysis. When an IV cannot be established, glucagon should be administered deep IM. There is a delay in therapeutic benefit because glucagon must first be absorbed and then act on target tissue in the liver to break down the stored form of glucose. Although the patient is not an insulin-dependent diabetic, she apparently has noninsulin-dependent diabetes mellitus based on the prescription of DiaBeta, an oral hypoglycemic agent. The presenting signs and symptoms are consistent with hypoglycemia.

134. (A) Insulin is secreted by the beta cells in the islets of Langerhans. Somatostatin is a hormone secreted by the delta cells. Although the role of somatostatin is not fully understood, it is believed to mediate the actions of both glucagon and insulin. Glycogenolysis is a function of glucagon intended to raise the blood glucose, while the action of insulin is to lower it. Insulin enhances the transfer of glucose into muscle and fat cells and is unnecessary for the transfer of glucose into brain cells.

135. (C) Thiamine is the treatment of choice for Wernicke's syndrome, a condition that results from long-term addiction to alcohol. The odor of ethanol (ETOH) and the circumstances suggest possible alcohol addiction. Chronic alcoholism can result in both nutritional deficiencies and impaired glucose metabolism. Thiamine (Vitamin B_1) is essential for glucose metabolism. If a bolus of glucose is administered to an alcoholic in the presence of Wernicke's syndrome, seizures may result due to the inability of the brain to metabolize glucose. $D_{50}W$ and naloxone are indicated to rule out hypoglycemia and narcotic overdose respectively, but should follow thiamine when ethanol addiction is suspected.

136. (A) The brain must receive a constant supply of glucose, since it cannot use fat or protein for fuel. Without this constant supply, brain cells will starve and cannot function properly. The resultant effects are the signs and symptoms associated with hypoglycemia, such as agitation, CNS stimulation followed by convulsions, and coma. Inadequate transport of glucose into the cells, inadequate synthesis of glycogen, and increased osmotic diuresis occur in the presence of too little insulin (hyperglycemia).

137. (B) In a 50-ml solution, half is glucose and half is water. By weight, there are 25 grams of glucose and 25 grams of water in this preloaded syringe.

138. (D) Physical findings indicate diabetic ketoacidosis (DKA) which is supported by the recent history of gastroenteritis associated with vomiting and diarrhea. Tachycardia and hypotension result from osmotic diuresis caused by an excessive serum glucose. Deep, rapid respirations (Kussmaul's respirations) are physiological attempts to correct the acidosis by eliminating both carbon dioxide and ketones. This information should lead to suspected DKA associated with the only elevated reagent reading listed.

139. (C) Oxygen is a medication and must always precede pharmaceuticals. Although it is tempting to immediately initiate an IV to administer parenteral agents, these efforts must never supersede 100% oxygen delivery to an unresponsive patient (except in the case of paraquat ingestion).

140. (A) Patients who have noninsulin-dependent diabetes mellitus (NIDDM) are at risk for a hyperglycemic derangement known as hyperosmolar coma. It differs from DKA in that it is not accompanied by acidosis. Glucatrol is one of several oral hypoglycemic agents prescribed to patients with NIDDM because it stimulates a poorly functioning pancreas to secrete insulin. Dehydration is the major risk factor for hyperosmolar coma. Patients predisposed to dehydration are the elderly and those taking diuretics. Decreased thirst mechanism and debility restricting access to fluid intake are common among the elderly. Diuretics produce additional loss. Central nervous system signs and symptoms may mimic a cerebrovascular accident but are caused by further dehydration due to osmotic diuresis associated with elevated serum glucose levels. Fluid resuscitation is necessary to correct hypovolemia, which results from severe dehydration.

141. (B) Because it is a hypertonic solution, $D_{50}W$ is very irritating to tissue. The IV must be started in a large vein where blood is circulated relatively rapidly (e.g., antecubital) to reduce possible phlebitis (inflammation of the vein) and infiltration. If infiltration occurs, administration must be immediately discontinued due to possible tissue necrosis and ultimate ulceration. $D_{50}W$ will not change the diameter of blood vessels nor produce ventricular ectopy. An elevated sensorium results from a successful response to administration.

142. (B) The brain stem is located at the base of the brain (inferior to the cerebellum) and contains the medulla and diencephalon. The medulla is the center for vital functions such as heart rate and respiratory activity. The diencephalon contains the thalamus (auditory and visual reflexes) and the hypothalamus (sleep-waking mechanisms, body temperature, hunger sensation, etc.). The cerebellum regulates muscular coordination and the constant awareness of an extremity's changing positions during movement (peripheral proprioception).

143. (D) The nervous system is divided into the central and peripheral nervous systems. The brain and spinal cord are subdivisions of the central

nervous system. The peripheral nervous system is divided into the sensory (afferent) and motor (efferent) nerves. Efferent nerves are functionally subdivided into voluntary and autonomic (involuntary) nerves.

144. (D) The medulla contains control centers for regulation of heartbeat, respirations, and blood pressure. The cerebrum is responsible for speech, memory, and thinking processes, and it includes the motor cortex, which controls voluntary motor activity, and the sensory cortex, which is responsible for interpretation of body sensations. The cerebellum coordinates muscle activity and maintains posture and equilibrium. The midbrain coordinates eye and head movements.

145. (D) The crossover of nerves occurs at the level of the medulla, that part of the brain stem to which the spinal cord is attached.

146. (C) The motor, verbal response, and eye opening parameters make up the Glasgow Coma Scale. Introduced in 1974, the scale has become a standard for describing level of consciousness.

147. (D) Altered LOC is the most important and significant change. Pupil changes are important, although they may be evidenced relatively late as intracranial pressure increases. The systolic blood pressure increases as the diastolic pressure decreases (widening pulse pressure) when intracranial pressure rises. The pulse rate also slows.

148. (B) Loss of sympathetic tone interferes with normal vasoconstriction needed to maintain blood pressure, and is the basis of neurogenic capacitance shock.

149. (A) A focal motor, or Jacksonian, seizure generally involves only one part of the body (face or arm). It is characterized by twitching that may start in the hand and then "marches" up the arm. This type of seizure may progress into a grand mal seizure, which is characterized by a loss of consciousness. As with any type of seizure, it is important to note where it started in order to aid the physician in determining the location of the irritable focus in the brain.

150. (D) There are many possible causes of seizure; therefore, it is important for the paramedic to obtain a thorough medical history on a patient experiencing a generalized motor seizure. Even when a known seizure

disorder is reported, the patient generally requires medical evaluation and should be transported to the hospital. Altered personality states occur with psychomotor seizures, not generalized motor seizures. Auras occur commonly with generalized motor seizures but are not always present.

151. (B) Status epilepticus is a medical emergency which requires rapid intervention to prevent serious complications or even death. Management differs from that of an isolated generalized motor seizure. Status epilepticus will usually benefit from field intervention. It is often caused by failure to take anticonvulsant medication.

152. (B) Protect the patient as much as possible from further injury or complications of seizure activity. A tongue blade is not used once a seizure has begun, because injury to the mouth and teeth can occur. Diazepam is used only if seizure activity continues without an intervening period of consciousness. Patients are never restrained, because this could cause soft tissue or skeletal injury.

153. (A) In addition to arteriosclerotic changes in the elderly, there are other causes of a CVA that may affect any age group. Many patients experience TIAs for some time prior to the CVA but may not seek medical attention. The degree of residual disability from the stroke varies from patient to patient.

154. (C) Field management of stroke includes oxygen at 6 liters, elevation of the head 15 degrees to facilitate venous drainage, and hyperventilation to reduce intracranial pressure if unresponsive. Corticosteroids are not indicated for the management of stroke. The Trendelenburg position is head down and feet elevated.

155. (C) Evaluation of neurologic status is sequential. The field neurologic exam provides a baseline of information. Repeated evaluations are important. The Glasgow Coma score is not intended to serve as the sole basis for therapy and is not the only factor evaluated in predicting survival. Deep tendon reflexes are not a routine part of the field neurologic exam.

156. (C) Vasoconstriction is a physiologic response that does not result from hypoventilation. Hypoventilation produces a rise in $PaCO_2$. This results

in vasodilatation that subsequently increases intracranial pressure. Hyperventilation decreases the $PaCO_2$, produces vasoconstriction, and reduces cerebral edema. Therefore, the patient with suspected increased intracranial pressure should be hyperventilated.

157. (D) Transient ischemic attacks (TIA) manifest as temporal neurologic deficits lasting less than 24 hours. The deficits often resolve within 15–60 minutes. After the attack, the patient does not demonstrate residual brain or neurologic damage. However, TIAs may forewarn of stroke. Embolic and thrombotic strokes leave residual neurologic signs and symptoms. Psychomotor seizures are focal seizures lasting 1–2 minutes.

158. (D) Personality and the motor center are located in the frontal lobe. The speech center is in the temporal lobe. Vision is located in the occipital lobe. Balance and coordination are a function of the cerebellum.

159. (B) During stress, the sympathetic division of the autonomic nervous system is dominant. Stimulation causes increases in heart rate, cardiac output, and blood pressure. It results in pupillary dilatation, bronchodilatation, and a rise in blood glucose. Parasympathetic stimulation is responsible for vegetative functions and produces the opposite effects. The brain and spinal cord comprise the central nervous system. The peripheral nervous system includes the cranial and peripheral nerves.

160. (A) Sodium bicarbonate should be administered to correct metabolic acidosis based on laboratory blood gas values. Naloxone is appropriate if narcotic overdose is suspected. Thiamine should be administered to suspected alcoholics. A steroid, such as dexamethasone, might be ordered if increased intracranial pressure is present. The pharmacological agents utilized for the comatose patient will vary according to local protocols.

161. (A) Field management of status epilepticus includes high flow oxygen with bag-valve-mask assistance to improve ventilation, diazepam to depress seizure activity, and dextrose 50% to treat hypoglycemia. Note that some EMS systems are using glucose only if a chemical reagent strip demonstrates that hypoglycemia is present. Tracheal intubation in the seizing patient is challenging and will probably require a paralyzing agent. Mannitol is used to reduce cerebral edema in closed head injury.

162. (B) Venous air embolism due to equipment or operator failure is a risk of hemodialysis. Acute onset of chest pain, respiratory distress, and cardiopulmonary arrest in this setting is highly suggestive of venous air embolism. The goal of placing the patient in a left, lateral position with the head lower than the legs is to trap the air bubble in the right atrium to prevent further embolism and complete blockage of the right ventricular outflow tract. Once this position has been achieved (referred to as Durant's maneuver), the primary assessment should proceed as usual. A tourniquet should never be applied to the extremity with a dialysis access site due to additional complications (including thrombosis, vascular insufficiency).

163. (C) Cholecystitis, or gallbladder inflammation, is classically characterized by the 6 Fs: female, fair, fat, forty, flatulent, and fertile. Although men and other women are not immune to gallbladder disease, the majority of patients with cholecystitis can typically be identified by the 6 Fs. Signs and symptoms of acute cholecystitis occur several hours after the patient's last meal. Excretion of bile occurs when fats are present because it emulsifies these large particles during digestion. The presence of stones in the gallbladder (cholelithiasis) impedes its ability to excrete bile into the duodenum and causes spasm resulting in pain. It is important to determine what the patient has eaten since a meal high in fatty or fried foods serves to support the diagnosis. A perforated ulcer presents with diffuse guarding and tenderness. Peptic ulcers do not result in RUQ discomfort. The acute onset of distress does not favor hepatitis as it is associated with a flu-like syndrome preceding more specific signs and symptoms.

164. (C) Diverticulitis is the inflammation of a thinned, pouched area (diverticulum) in the large intestine. A diverticulum is usually caused by chronic constipation or poor elimination habits. The pouch continues to collect stool, becomes infected, and may rupture similar to an aneurysm. Feces and bacteria then spill into the peritoneal cavity. Irritation may result in localized peritonitis while rupture causes generalized peritonitis. Diverticulitis usually involves the rectum causing LLQ pain and tenderness.

165. (C) A renal calculus, or kidney stone, which obstructs urine outflow from the kidney to the bladder, causes extreme pain. The location of pain depends on the location of the stone within the outflow tract and

the area of obstruction. A history of hematuria, or blood in the urine, supports your suspicion. Differentiating renal calculi from peritonitis is not difficult. Patients with kidney stone pain present with "walking colic." They are extremely restless, seeking a position of comfort that is unattainable until the stone has passed or is removed. The patient with peritonitis does not move because movement aggravates the pain. The patient lies perfectly still, usually with knees flexed to prevent tension on the peritoneum. Appendicitis, ruptured diverticulum, and perforated viscus (organ) present with some degree of peritoneal irritation.

166. (A) In order to prevent guarding, it is important to assess the region of complaint last. Assessment should begin with the opposite area, the RLQ in this case, and proceed clockwise with the painful region last. Otherwise, the patient will tense the abdominal muscles (voluntary guarding) or reflex abdominal muscle contraction will occur (involuntary guarding). This will make it virtually impossible to assess the abdomen.

167. (B) The most characteristic physical finding of an abdominal aneurysm is a pulsating mass. Once the mass is detected, cease palpation of the abdomen. Extensive palpation may cause the aneurysm to rupture. Peritonitis presents with a rigid abdominal wall with rebound tenderness and possible absent bowel sounds. A ruptured spleen is most often secondary to trauma in the upper left quadrant. The classic signs of appendicitis are tenderness and muscle spasm in the right lower quadrant.

168. (B) Testicular torsion results from a congenital defect of the spermatic cord. It is referred to as a bell-clapper deformity because the testicle is suspended from the spermatic cord like the clapper of a bell. When the cord is too long, there is sufficient slack to allow excessive movement of the testicle within the scrotum. The cord eventually becomes twisted, causing testicular vascular insufficiency. This condition usually appears immediately preceding or following the onset of puberty. It is considered an emergency because the testicle will become necrotic requiring surgical removal if not treated within a few hours.

169. (D) The clear catheter originating from the periumbilical area is consistent with a peritoneal dialysis device. Continuous ambulatory peritoneal dialysis (CAPD) is the machine-free method of accomplishing renal dialysis when 95% of renal function has been lost due to end-stage

renal disease (ESRD). Using the peritoneal membrane as a filter, dialysis solution is introduced into the peritoneal cavity by a surgically implanted catheter. After a predetermined amount of time, the solution is removed and fresh dialyzing fluid is infused. The catheter is clamped and the process begins again. Insulin-dependent diabetes mellitus (IDDM) should be suspected because it is the leading cause of ESRD. Insulin can be mixed into the dialysis solution for continuous absorption across the peritoneal membrane. Therefore, you must also assume hypoglycemia and manage the case accordingly.

170. (D) Melena (black, tarry stool) and hematemesis (vomiting blood) are signs of gastrointestinal bleeding. Vital signs and physical findings indicate critical blood loss with hypovolemic shock. Dopamine is contraindicated in the presence of inadequate circulating volume. If hypotension and physical findings do not improve after adequate fluid resuscitation, dopamine can be used for possible cardiogenic shock. Fluid resuscitation and oxygen administration are indicated in this situation. Due to the patient's complaint of nausea and history of vomiting, it is doubtful if he can tolerate oxygen adjuncts other than the cannula. Although not ideal, the cannula will enhance the FiO_2 (percentage of inspired oxygen). The pneumatic antishock garment may be utilized according to local protocol.

171. (B) Oxygen administration and ECG monitoring are appropriate. Fluid resuscitation may be indicated using normal saline. Although renal failure causes retention of both sodium and potassium, toxic effects of hyperkalemia (excessive potassium) on cardiac function preclude the administration of fluid containing potassium, such as lactated Ringer's. Hypovolemia is typically encountered during dialysis rather than after the procedure. Postural hypotension with syncope is not uncommon following dialysis because excess fluids that accumulate prior to dialysis are removed. Dopamine is not indicated in this scenario.

172. (D) Sensitization involves the production of antibodies that attach to mast cells. Following sensitization, contact with an antigen results in the attachment of an antigen to antibodies on the mast cells. This causes the mast cells to release histamine and heparin. The release of histamine results in bronchoconstriction, vasodilation, and increased capillary permeability. Signs and symptoms of anaphylaxis result largely from the effects of histamine.

173. (A) Epinephrine 0.5 mg SQ is the maximum adult dose of the first drug of choice to correct an anaphylactic reaction. Its antihistamine actions result from an ability to stop the mast cells from releasing histamine.

174. (D) Aminophylline promotes relaxation of smooth muscle in the tracheobronchial tree resulting in bronchodilatation. During anaphylaxis, histamine is released from mast cells causing smooth muscle constriction. Other anaphylactic substances cause increased capillary permeability resulting in edema. Edema results in additional bronchospasm.

175. (C) Poor peripheral perfusion due to vasodilation during anaphylaxis necessitates deep intramuscular (IM) injection. Due to the sedating effects of Benadryl causing possible respiratory depression, rapid IV administration is not desirable. The chemical composition could cause tissue damage, and therefore, is not appropriate for subcutaneous (SQ) administration.

176. (B) Vomiting should not be induced in a patient who has ingested caustic substances, or is in an unconscious state. Protection of the airway has priority in the treatment of this patient, therefore, the airway should be protected with an endotracheal tube as soon as possible. Starting an intravenous infusion with D_5W maintains a lifeline to administer medications as needed. Definitive treatment needs to be initiated at an appropriate hospital, and transportation should begin as soon as possible.

177. (B) Oxygen administration is contraindicated in cases of paraquat ingestion. Once absorbed into the circulation, paraquat forms a radical in the alveoli which oxidizes when exposed to oxygen. This causes irreversible and extensive damage to these structures. Oxygen administration is indicated after arterial blood gases are obtained and the pO_2 is determined to be markedly decreased. Paraquat ingestion is the only true contraindication for oxygen administration.

178. (B) The need to increase the dosage of drugs to achieve the same effect is called tolerance. Psychologic dependence is the need to use a drug to maintain support of the psyche, i.e., emotional state of well-being. Physical dependence and addiction are the physiologic need to use a drug to avoid the symptoms of withdrawal.

179. (C) Cyanide is used in many electroplating processes. This patient presents with some of the signs and symptoms associated with cyanide poisoning. Amyl nitrite is the first drug given because it stops the toxic process by disengaging cyanide from hemoglobin. Oxygen administration will be ineffective initially because hemoglobin bound to cyanide does not have a site available for oxygen. Once inhalation of amyl nitrite spirits has been initiated, oxygen therapy is begun. IV sodium thiosulfate follows IV sodium nitrite, which is given after discontinuing amyl nitrite. Fifty percent dextrose in water will not correct the problem and will delay definitive treatment.

180. (B) The signs, symptoms, and assessment findings are consistent with serious salicylate toxicity. Sodium bicarbonate should be administered to counteract the metabolic acidosis that develops rapidly following an overdose. Syrup of ipecac is not indicated due to the extended period of elapsed time. Activated charcoal could be administered, but this should be done via nasogastric tube due to the respiratory distress and potential for aspiration.

181. (B) Envenomization by a brown recluse spider (or fiddler spider) is generally painless. After 2–3 days, however, effects from the venom become apparent. A reddened area encircled by dark, necrotic tissue appears. In the past, treatment required surgical excision of the lesion and skin grafts. Dapsone (a medication used to treat leprosy) has proven effective in treating the wound without surgery. Pit viper and scorpion envenomizations are accompanied by immediate pain and edema. Venom from a black widow spider does not cause tissue necrosis. Mild to severe muscle cramping with possible tetany are the primary complaints associated with black widow spider envenomization.

182. (A) Imipramine (trade name, Tofranil) is a family of tricyclic antidepressants (TCA). A toxic effect of TCA is an increased QRS duration as shown on the ECG. TCAs are protein-bound drugs that have a long half-life. Increasing the blood pH with sodium bicarbonate to alkaline levels enhances protein binding, which decreases the amount of free-drug. Less free-drug means there are fewer pharmacological effects. Physostigmine is a direct antidote for anticholinergic toxicity but carries a high risk of inducing ventricular fibrillation in this setting. Quinidine is contraindicated because its cardiovascular actions are similar to those of TCA.

183. (C) Since the most likely problem is organophosphate poisoning, the drug of choice is atropine sulfate. Organophosphates are cholinergic insecticides. SLUDGE is the mnemonic for typical signs and symptoms: Salivation, Lacrimation, Urination, Defecation, Gastric discomfort, Emesis. Atropine produces anticholinergic effects. The initial dose is 2.0 mg, which is repeated until secretions begin to dry or excessive tachycardia develops.

184. (C) Seconal is a bright red barbiturate capsule prescribed as a sleeping pill. Signs and symptoms consistent with barbiturate toxicity include decreased LOC, bradypnea, and widely dilated pupils. Cocaine is a CNS stimulant. Heroin is ineffective when ingested. Phencyclidine is a sympathomimetic analgesic which causes CNS stimulation and psychoses.

185. (A) Application of cold packs is contraindicated in the management of snake bite because it increases tissue damage. Immobilization of the limb decreases discomfort and delays absorption. Crystalloid IV fluids should be initiated to treat potential hypotension. A constricting band placed above the site of envenomization assists in decreasing the rate of venom absorption. This is a constricting band only, not a tourniquet.

186. (B) The setting of an automotive workshop with poor ventilation creates a high index of suspicion for excessive accumulations of carbon monoxide. When several people who share the workshop environment present with generalized, nonspecific complaints, you should suspect carbon monoxide poisoning. Their symptoms are due to hypoxia because carbon monoxide tightly binds to hemoglobin. Soon, there are no sites on the hemoglobin for oxygen binding to occur. Chlorine and ammonia inhalations are associated with tracheobronchial burns and pain. Aromatic benzenes (e.g., paint propellant) have an odor that would be detectable on your arrival.

187. (B) DTs (delirium tremens) occur within 48–72 hours after the patient stops drinking. As the blood alcohol returns to normal (0), physical effects of withdrawal are seen. These include tremors, seizures, anxiety, and psychological disturbances such as hallucinations.

188. (D) Ethanol inhibits the metabolism of wood alcohol and promotes its elimination. Syrup of ipecac would not be indicated because the patient is unresponsive. A nasogastric tube would be required for activated char-

coal administration. Ethylene glycol is antifreeze and contraindicated for ingestion.

189. (A) The T-lymphocyte system has two major components: T-helpers and T-suppressors. T-helper lymphocytes attack the foreign invader in an effort to destroy it. T-suppressor lymphocytes are normally present in fewer numbers than T-helpers. They become involved in the immune response to bring the "war" to a close. When HIV infects a T-helper cell, it uses the T-helper's DNA to reproduce itself. This results in T-helper destruction and lowers their numbers to less than T-suppressors. In this case, the immune response not only becomes less effective due to decreased T-helpers but also inhibited due to a higher ratio of T-suppressors to T-helpers. B-lymphocytes produce the circulating antibodies referred to as immunoglobulins.

190. (C) Meningococcal meningitis is a bacterial infection involving the central nervous system. This child has signs consistent with meningococcemia, i.e., pinpoint subcutaneous hemorrhagic lesions, or petechiae. Nuchal rigidity (inability to flex the head in chin-to-chest maneuver) indicates the presence of meningeal irritation. This is a highly communicable disease that is spread by airborne droplets. Prophylaxis of all individuals having contact with the patient will be required.

191. (A) Prehospital care providers routinely come in contact with blood during BLS and ALS procedures. If the EMS provider has open cuts or skin lesions, contamination by the patient's blood can occur. The droplet mode, including saliva, is not known to spread the HIV virus.

192. (B) AIDS is the diagnosis when the HIV+ patient develops pathology consistent with immune deficiency (e.g., Karposi's sarcoma, pneumocystis carinii, etc.). AIDS related complex (ARC) is a condition that may be identified in the early stages of acquired immune deficiency. It is defined as a variety of signs and symptoms associated with immunosuppression (e.g., unexplained weight loss of 10 pounds or more; night sweats; candidiasis; chronic diarrhea; etc.) together with a positive test for Human Immunodeficiency Virus (HIV+). Patients who are taking immunosuppressive drugs following chemotherapy or organ transplantation are immunosuppressed but not HIV+.

193. (C) Isoniazid is a medication used in the treatment of tuberculosis (TB). Signs and symptoms characteristic of active TB include pleuritic pain,

productive cough, fever that spikes at night causing diaphoresis, and abdominal pain due to referral and/or coughing. The thin, emaciated appearance is due to the high metabolic demands associated with the disease and is the basis for its old name—consumption. TB is spread by respiratory droplet and is highly contagious. Isoniazid rules out pneumonia, pneumocystis, and immune deficiency. Pneumocystis carinii is an infection seen only in patients with immune deficiency. It should be noted that TB has become more prevalent over the past few years due to increasing numbers of homeless shelters and AIDS cases. TB spreads easily among close contacts over a period of a few months. It is also seen with HIV+ cases due to impaired T-lymphocytes which are responsible for attacking normally slow-developing infections such as TB.

194. (D) Herpes zoster is a viral condition referred to as shingles. The chickenpox virus (varicella zoster) lies dormant in nerve endings that follow the spinal tract dermatomes. In some individuals, blisters reoccur along a dermatome months or years after active chickenpox has resolved. Shingles usually appear when the individual has been under stress. Stress causes immune suppression resulting from increased secretion of adrenal corticosteroids. Although shingles cannot be transmitted, anyone who has not had chickenpox can acquire this disease from weeping shingle lesions which contain the virus. Although there is no cure for either shingles or chickenpox, Vesicular Immune Globulin (VZIG) may be given prophylactically to individuals who have not had chickenpox and have been exposed to the virus.

195. (B) All viruses, including the delta hepatitis virus, contain only RNA and are not capable of reproducing without a host organism. Delta hepatitis virus, in addition to host DNA, requires Hepatitis B virus (HBV) to reproduce. The patient with delta hepatitis must have HBV present, even if asymptomatic during HBV infection. HAV causes inflammation of the liver and is communicated by the fecal/oral route. HCV was formerly classified as hepatitis nonA-nonB (NANB, not type A or type B) because the virus had not been isolated. This disease is contracted by direct contact with blood or through transfusion. Hepatitis NANB remains a category because it is believed that other hepatitis viruses have yet to be isolated.

196. (B) Any agent capable of destroying tuberculosis bacteria is capable of destroying other bacteria as well as HIV and HBV. These types of disinfectants are used by hospitals and display this information on their la-

bels. Alcohol and Betadine iodine are ineffective against most bacteria and viruses as a disinfectant. One-part bleach and ten-part water solution is also effective. A bleach solution of 1:100 is too dilute and will be ineffective.

197. (A) The presence of scleral jaundice (icterus) indicates liver involvement. Hepatitis A virus (HAV) is usually contracted by eating contaminated food and is spread by fecal-oral contamination. Typical causes include raw shellfish from polluted water, contaminated drinking water, and poor hygiene by infected individuals in the food service industry. Following an incubation period of 25–40 days, an infected person develops a viral syndrome (flu-like signs and symptoms) and jaundice. Unlike HBV infection, HAV resolves itself and is not transmitted after the infection has passed. Permanent liver damage and serious complications are possible with HAV infection, but are less common than with HBV. An acute abdomen is characterized by peritonitis. Bloody diarrhea is associated with salmonella infection. Gastroenteritis does not cause jaundice.

198. (C) Pneumomediastinum is a pulmonary overpressure accident that may occur during rapid ascent, if the diver holds his breath during ascent, or if there is predisposition to rupture due to pulmonary blebs. Rupture may occur during ascent because pulmonary gases expand at this time. Pneumomediastinum occurs when the rupture releases gas through the visceral pleura into the mediastinum and/or pericardial sac. Mechanism of injury produces a high index of suspicion. Signs and symptoms consistent with pneumomediastinum include substernal pain, change in voice quality, irregular pulse, hypotension, narrow pulse pressure, abnormal heart sounds, and possible mild cyanosis. Hemopericardium results from myocardial injury or disruption. Neither tension pneumothorax, hemopericardium, nor venous air embolism affects voice quality.

199. (A) Heat exhaustion occurs when a hot environment induces salt and fluid loss due to excessive perspiration. Signs and symptoms include weakness, vertigo, nausea, syncope, pallor, diaphoresis, and tachycardia. The blood pressure may be elevated or decreased depending on the amount of fluid that has been lost. Heat cramps, as the name implies, is associated with painful spasms of fingers, arms, legs, and/or abdominal muscles. Heat stroke would not be suspected in this case because the patient regained consciousness after the syncopal episode.

200. (A) Cervical spine injury must always be suspected in cases of diving injuries. Since the modified jaw thrust does not involve repositioning the head, it is the most appropriate manual maneuver to establish an open airway. The triple airway maneuver involves head-tilt, jaw thrust, and chin-lift.

201. (D) Movement of the severely hypothermic patient can stimulate the return of cool extremity blood and acids to the core, resulting in a decrease of the core temperature or "after-drop." This cold, acidotic blood causes cardiac dysrhythmias including ventricular fibrillation. Cellular metabolic needs do not increase until the core temperature has been raised.

202. (C) This patient presents with signs indicating a core temperature of <90°F (severe hypothermia). Atrial fibrillation with a slow ventricular response is the most common dysrhythmia associated with severe hypothermia when the patient has a pulse. Heart and respiratory rates are sufficient to meet the significantly reduced metabolic needs during this state. Therefore, the patient should be moved gently and transported quickly but carefully to the hospital for rewarming. Stimulation with intubation or ventilation usually results in the development of ventricular fibrillation. Infusing IV fluids will further reduce the core temperature due to the after-drop phenomenon or IV fluid temperature.

203. (B) Blood vessels in the extremities are constricted as the body attempts to prevent unnecessary heat loss from nonessential areas. Heat application to the extremities causes vasodilation with subsequent return of cold, acidotic blood to the core. Large blood vessels lie superficially in the head, neck, lateral chest wall, and groin. Application of heat in these areas will assist in returning warm blood to the core.

204. (B) The ECG demonstrates ventricular fibrillation. Although local protocol may vary, the DOT curriculum recommends an initial defibrillation of 400J after initiating CPR. Repeated defibrillation is then recommended only if the core temperature is ≥85°F. The initial dose of lidocaine is 1 mg/kg but should be repeated every 15 minutes at 0.5 mg/kg (maximum 3 mg/kg) to prevent toxicity due to inadequate drug metabolism in the presence of hypothermia. Rewarming is attempted if the ETA is more than 15 minutes. Endotracheal intubation and ventilation are indicated in the management of ventricular fibrillation. However, the oxygen must be warmed to >99°F to prevent de-

creasing the core temperature any further. **This represents the recommendations from the DOT curriculum. You must follow your local protocol in the actual clinical setting.**

205. (D) The body produces heat by shivering. This is counterproductive to your objective of reducing body temperature.

206. (A) Beta particles have slightly more penetrating energy than Alpha particles. They are similar to Alpha particles in that serious damage may result from inhalation or ingestion.

207. (C) When the face and nose are subjected to cold water, a series of events occur that are collectively referred to as the "diving reflex" or "mammalian diving reflex." Respiration is inhibited, heart rate slows, and systemic blood vessels constrict, decreasing blood flow to all tissues except for cerebral and myocardial. Oxygen is delivered only to those tissues that are essential for survival. As the temperature of the water decreases, the amount of oxygen flow to the brain and heart increases. Decreased metabolism and hypothermia aid in preventing additional cellular destruction but do not prioritize oxygen delivery. Laryngospasm is an airway protective mechanism that contributes to asphyxiation.

208. (D) Transient Ischemic Attacks (TIA) are episodes of focal cerebral dysfunction that last minutes or occasionally up to an hour. They differ from cerebrovascular accidents (CVA) in that neurological deficits do not persist for more than 24 hours. Neither acute myocardial infarction (AMI) nor DKA (diabetic ketoacidosis) produce focal weakness or eyelid drooping, ptosis.

209. (C) Peripheral edema may be caused by varicose veins, inactivity, and position, and is not always a sign of congestive heart failure. Jugular venous distention (JVD) is significant if present when the patient's head is elevated 45°. Any patient who complains of severe dyspnea, regardless of age, is presumed to be hypoxic and must be treated. The elderly may also have nonpathological rales.

210. (A) Elderly persons are more prone to head injury, even from relatively minor trauma as in this scenario. This is due to a significant difference in proportion between the brain and skull. Signs of brain compression may develop more slowly, sometimes over days or weeks. In these situations, the patient may even forget having an accident. A subdural

hematoma is bleeding that takes place below the dura. It develops more slowly than an epidural hematoma because a subdural generally involves venous bleeding. Disrupted meningeal arteries are usually responsible for an epidural hematoma.

211. (A) A general decline in organ systems occurs with aging. Normal left ventricular hypertrophy (enlargement) is up to 25%, not 45%.

212. (A) In the elderly, edema in the lower extremities is often related to inactivity or sitting with the feet dependent. Edema subsides with movement or elevation of the extremity. Edema of the lower extremities resulting from chronic congestive heart failure does not subside with elevation of the affected part. Right-sided ventricular failure produces neck vein distention. The patient with pulmonary edema presents with dyspnea and rales.

213. (D) Mr. Fleming is suffering from an acute hypertensive crisis. Quadriplegia, or paralysis of all four extremities, results from spinal cord disruption. He could, however, present with hemiplegia (paralysis of one-half of the body). Hemiparesis is weakness of either the right or left half of the body. Ataxic (uncoordinated) gait and disorientation can result from acute hypertensive crisis due to inadequate cerebral perfusion.

214. (A) The ECG is sinus rhythm with bigeminal PVCs. Acute suppressive therapy with lidocaine is indicated in this setting. Even though the patient is not over 70 years of age, the dosage must be reduced by 50% because he has signs and symptoms consistent with congestive heart failure. Lidocaine metabolism is primarily accomplished in the liver. Hepatic blood flow is significantly reduced with right ventricular failure as increased pressure from the heart is quickly reflected into the inferior vena cava.

215. (B) Declining function of organs and systems occurs with aging. The temperature declines due to decreased hypothalmic ability, diminished cardiac output, loss of subcutaneous tissue, decreased shivering capability, and decreased metabolism. Overall, the body does not require as much energy and, therefore, produces less heat. The decline in depth of subcutaneous tissue not only produces poor skin turgor but also results in a loss of insulation to preserve the heat that is produced. A geriatric patient with a rectal temperature of 99°F is considered to have a febrile process until proven otherwise.

216. (C) Senile dementia of the Alzheimer's type is a chronic, progressive, and degenerative disease that affects the brain. It results in the destruction of cognitive abilities. Behavior ranges from inappropriate to raging outbursts.

217. (B) This patient has taken an overdose of a tricyclic antidepressant (TCA). TCA intoxication can rapidly produce unconsciousness without warning. Therefore, emetic medications such as syrup of ipecac should never be given in this setting. Alkalizing the blood with either sodium bicarbonate or hyperventilation decreases the quantity of circulating active drug and its effects. Tracheal intubation by either the nasal or oral routes may be necessary if the patient becomes unresponsive. This was apparently a suicide gesture. Suicide is the fourth leading cause of death in the elderly.

218. (B) A hot, humid environment without an evaporation gradient renders the body's ability to cool itself through the sweating mechanism ineffective. This allows the core temperature to rise, causing increased metabolism. Loss of body fluid and electrolytes decreases blood volume as perspiration continues to be produced in a futile effort to cool the core. As the temperature continues to rise, generalized vasodilation leads to complete cardiovascular collapse. Cellular necrosis occurs as well. Heat stroke is suspected when there is a history of exposure to a hot and humid (>75%) environment together with decreased LOC, flushed or wet skin, tachycardia (early) or bradycardia (late), hypotension, low diastolic pressure, and tachypnea (early) or bradypnea (late). Fluid resuscitation is necessary to replace circulating volume, facilitate cooling of the core, and prevent cardiovascular collapse. One to two IVs of normal saline or lactated Ringer's should be started and administered at a wide open rate.

219. (D) External compression is the best method for controlling a child's simple, unilateral nose bleed. This is generally achieved by pinching the nostrils together. Hemostats are not used in the field to control bleeding. External compression will be more effective than application of ice. Packing the nose is not recommended in the field.

220. (B) Especially after an accident, the young child's normal fear of separation is heightened by worry that something terrible has happened to the parents.

221. (B) The age of the sick or injured child will determine your basic approach. Infants must be approached differently than toddlers, and toddlers require a different approach than an older child. The correct approach will help you to gain the child's cooperation.

222. (D) Nuchal rigidity, or stiffness of the neck, is a common finding in meningitis (an infection involving the tissues covering the brain and spinal cord). Meningitis is a serious illness with potentially lethal complications. Vomiting is common with most infants and many older children with most illnesses or injuries, regardless of severity. A fever of 103°F may be common with even a relatively mild illness. Pulsation of the anterior fontanelle is a normal finding.

223. (B) The most common response of the newborn to hypoxia is bradycardia. In older children, tachycardia is the first response. Other rhythm disturbances such as premature ventricular or atrial contractions may occur, but are not common consequences of hypoxia.

224. (B) Asthma results in bronchoconstriction that produces edema, congestion, and wheezing. This condition affects mainly the expiratory phase of respiration. Bronchiolitis is an inflammation caused by a virus and is not a chronic condition. A good history will help you determine whether the patient has bronchiolitis or asthma. Epiglottitis and croup are diseases that affect the upper airway.

225. (B) The appropriate treatment for a patient with an acute asthma attack should include oxygen administration to treat hypoxia and bronchodilator therapy, such as albuterol or terbutaline via nebulizer. Parenteral beta-agonists are less effective than inhaled therapy. An IV route may be considered if the patient is in respiratory failure or requires rehydration. Epinephrine 1:10,000 is used in cardiac arrest situations and is not appropriate in the treatment of asthma.

226. (C) The dosage of epinephrine 1:1000 calculated by weight is 0.01 ml/kg, which, for a 15 kg child, would be 0.15 ml.

227. (D) Most cases of laryngotracheobronchitis (croup) respond to the administration of humidified oxygen. The patient should be kept in a sitting position and transported in the company of a parent. Severe cases of croup may require administration of racemic epinephrine by

nebulizer. Subcutaneous epinephrine is not a management protocol for croup. The paramedic should not visualize the upper airway of a child with stridor.

228. (C) Bronchiolitis is a viral disease most often affecting children between the ages of 2 months and 2 years. Lower airway obstruction is due to inflammation and mucus collection rather than bronchospasm. Asthma generally affects children over 2 years of age and is frequently due to an allergy. Signs and symptoms of croup include barking cough and loud stridor. Pneumonia presents with high fever, productive cough, and segmental lung consolidation.

229. (A) Epiglottitis usually occurs in children over the age of 4 and is characterized by pain on swallowing, drooling, and a high temperature. Croup more commonly affects children under 4 and is characterized by inspiratory stridor and a seal-like bark.

230. (D) Allow the child to assume the position of greatest comfort. Forcing a reclining position can aggravate the child and cause crying. This will complicate the respiratory problem. The tripod-type position allows for the fullest expansion of the chest wall and is the position frequently chosen.

231. (B) The healthy child can usually tolerate dysrhythmias better than the adult patient, and therefore aggressive treatment may not be indicated. Anemia results in sinus tachycardia. Occasional PVCs are not uncommon in children and generally do not require treatment. PSVT often terminates without therapy and is usually well tolerated.

232. (C) Trauma is the leading cause of death in children over 3 years of age. Trauma results from automobile and other types of accidents, including falls, abuse, and burns. While deaths that are associated with congenital disorders, seizures, and meningitis do occur, most deaths in this age group are trauma-related.

233. (C) Children are more susceptible than adults to seizures associated with an elevated temperature. Seizures may occur with equal frequency resulting from head injury, toxic ingestion, and hypoxia in both children and adults.

234. (D) Common autopsy findings that help confirm the diagnosis of SIDS include intrathoracic petechiae, pulmonary congestion and edema, and

aspiration of gastric contents (a terminal event). Pneumonia and septicemia rule out a diagnosis of SIDS.

235. (B) SIDS cannot be predicted or prevented. The etiology is unknown. SIDS is not the result of either child abuse or suffocation.

236. (C) A simple laceration with no other signs of injury is seen quite commonly in children who have fallen forward and hit their chins against unforgiving objects. Take a history! A minor, first-time injury, with a logical history of incident, would not usually lead you to suspect child abuse. If the child has made frequent trips to EDs in the area, is described by the attending adult as "accident prone," or has siblings with recent histories of major injuries, you should report suspected child abuse. Be alert to burns that do not fit the history offered; a 2-year-old who pulls a cup of coffee off a table does not sustain partial and full-thickness burns over 35% of the body.

237. (C) The educational level of the abusive parent is not a significant factor in child abuse. However, abuse is found more frequently in lower socioeconomic groups, related to poor living conditions, unemployment, etc. The abuser frequently feels isolated, unworthy (low self-esteem), and lacks resources or feels unable to seek assistance. Expectations of the child are frequently unrealistic and rigid.

238. (A) Primary cardiac problems occur with less frequency in children than airway obstruction, CNS depression or injury, near-drowning, or shock. The paramedic should suspect causes other than cardiac problems in the child experiencing cardiopulmonary arrest. Obstruction of the airway by a foreign object is a common occurrence in a young child.

239. (B) The standard compression rate for children is 80–100 compressions per minute. The compression rate for children is 80 per minute and for infants is 100 per minute. These rates should provide the needed circulation, but allow time for adequate cardiac filling.

240. (D) Abdominal thrusts should not be performed in infants or young children, because of the possibility of damage to the liver and other intra-abdominal organs. Back blows may be effective in dislodging a foreign body. Chest thrusts may also be used and are performed like external chest compressions. The paramedic should open the mouth to inspect for foreign objects, but should *not* perform blind sweeps since a foreign body may be pushed back and cause further obstruction.

241. (B) The correct initial dose to defibrillate infants and children is 2 joules/kg. If this is unsuccessful, the initial dose should be doubled. If this is ineffective, acid/base balance and oxygenation should be reassessed.

242. (B) The correct pediatric dosage of epinephrine is 0.10 ml/kg, 1:10,000 solution or 0.01 mg/kg. While many drug dosages are given in mg/kg, at the present time all current references for epinephrine are ml/kg. Solutions of 1:1000 should not be used for management of cardiac arrest.

243. (C) The correct dosage of atropine for a pediatric patient is 0.01–0.02 mg/kg. This patient weighs 15 kg (33 pounds); therefore, 0.2 mg is an appropriate dosage.

244. (A) Bronchiolitis is an inflammation of the bronchioles caused by a viral infection in children under 2 years of age and does not affect the upper airway. Laryngotracheobronchitis and epiglottitis may both produce symptoms of upper airway obstruction and must be differentiated from foreign body obstruction.

245. (C) The blood pressure cuff for the pediatric patient should cover two-thirds of the upper arm.

246. (C) Intravenous fluids should be initiated at 20 ml/kg. The patient should be evaluated after the fluid bolus and may need to receive an additional bolus(es) titrated to the clinical response. Fluid administration must always be monitored closely in children to prevent overload.

247. (B) As a rule, a cuffed endotracheal tube is used in children over 8 years of age. In children less than 8 years, the circular narrowing at the level of the cricoid cartilage serves as a functional cuff. A properly selected uncuffed tube will allow for a minimal air leak at the cricoid ring.

248. (B) It is important to remember that the glottis in the infant is higher in the neck than the adult. There are other anatomical differences in the anatomy and size of the infant vs. adult airways. The tongue of the infant is larger in relation to the other surrounding structures, and the vocal cords slant upward and backward.

249. (A) Endotracheal intubation is appropriate in the young child. The esophageal obturator airway is not recommended because various

esophageal tube lengths and face mask sizes are required. Nasotracheal intubation may be required post-admission when long-term ventilatory support is required. However, passage of a nasotracheal tube or nasopharyngeal airway may be difficult and result in bleeding from enlarged adenoidal tissue. Cricothyrotomy is not recommended in children less than 8 years of age due to difficulty in establishing landmarks. The cricoid area is also the narrowest segment of the airway. Oxygen-powered breathing devices are not recommended due to the risk of gastric distention and tension pneumothorax.

250. (C) The primary purposes of the pediatric IV calibrated volume set are delivery of small, measured quantities of fluid and the prevention of runaway IVs. The sets are also utilized when a measured amount of medication is to be delivered over a given period of time. The sets provide no filtering function.

251. (D) The first choice for intraosseous cannulation is 1–3 centimeters below the tibial tuberosity. Only one attempt can be made in each bone. The second preferred site is the femur.

252. (D) You should attempt to gain the child's cooperation by being honest and acknowledging when a procedure will be painful. Give the child permission to cry. An ill or injured preschooler is not feeling brave, but vulnerable and out of control. Parents should be included in the child's care when appropriate, by holding the IV bag, holding the child's hand, etc. This will decrease both the child's and parent's anxiety. Explain in simple terms what you are doing. Remember that some common words or phrases may be frightening to a child. The child may wonder where you are going to "take" his or her blood pressure to.

253. (B) Due to generally excellent vascular tone, supine blood pressure may remain normal with a blood loss of 20–25%. Therefore, a drop in blood pressure is a late sign, and may occur much later than in the adult patient. If hypovolemia is suspected, and supine vital signs are normal, orthostatic vital signs are appropriate. Capillary refill should be evaluated frequently and may indicate hypovolemia before vital sign changes occur.

254. (B) In the infant and child, the 5:1 compression-ventilation ratio is maintained for both one and two rescuers. A pause of 1 to 1.5 seconds should occur after the fifth compression to permit adequate ventilation.

255. (C) The correct initial dosage of sodium bicarbonate for the pediatric patient, as for the adult, is 1 mEq/kg. In this situation, the patient should receive 12 mEq.

256. (B) Bradycardia in infants is a heart rate of less than 80 beats per minute. Bradycardia usually results from hypoxia.

257. (D) In infants under 1 year of age, the brachial or femoral arteries are recommended to assess the pulse. Over 1 year of age, the carotid is recommended. The carotid is difficult to palpate in the chubby neck of the infant. The radial artery is less central and may also be difficult to find in the infant. The apical impulse is not a pulse and its absence does not correlate with absence of cardiac activity.

258. (D) Cardiac arrest in children is not a sudden event. It is usually an end result of progressive deterioration in respiratory and circulatory failure. Cardiac arrest can often be prevented by early recognition of symptoms of respiratory failure and prompt initiation of treatment.

259. (A) Atropine, epinephrine, and lidocaine may all be administered via the endotracheal route. Sodium bicarbonate and calcium are sclerosing to small veins and can produce chemical burns.

260. (D) This child is at risk for dehydration. A sunken fontanelle is seen in moderate to severe dehydration. The respiratory and pulse rates are normal for this age. Mottling of the extremities when crying is normal in the newborn.

6

OB/GYN and Neonatal

1. Functions of the placenta include which of the following?

    (1) Storage mechanism for nutrients.
    (2) Excretion of CO_2 and waste products.
    (3) Transfer of oxygen and nutrients.
    (4) Production of hormones to maintain pregnancy.
    (5) Transfer of antibodies.

  A. 2, 3, 5.
  B. 1, 2, 3, 5.
  C. 2, 3, 4, 5.
  D. 1, 2, 3, 4.

2. Your patient is a 24-year-old sexually active female. She is complaining of severe RLQ and LLQ pain. She states that she has had a heavy yellow vaginal discharge for three weeks and has had a history of irregular menses. Vital signs are within normal limits. You suspect this patient has:

  A. Renal calculus.
  B. Amenorrhea.
  C. BSO.
  D. PID.

3. Fertilization normally occurs in the:

  A. Fallopian tubes.
  B. Endometrium.
  C. Uterus.
  D. Vagina.

4. If indicated, when should you add oxytocin to an IV?

  A. At the end of the second stage of labor.
  B. During the last stage of labor.
  C. At the end of the third stage of labor.
  D. During the first stage of labor.

5. A 19-year-old female is complaining of severe left shoulder pain. She is cold, pale, clammy, and apprehensive. There is minimal pink vaginal discharge. You would suspect:

A. Pelvic inflammatory disease.
B. Ruptured ectopic pregnancy.
C. Dysmenorrhea.
D. Salpingitis.

6. Your patient is a 25-year-old (gravida 1, para 0) who called EMS because she thinks labor has started. During the physical examination, you learn that her expected due date is two months from now. When assessing her discomfort, you learn the contractions are worse while lying still and are eased by walking. This clinical picture is consistent with which of the following?

A. Braxton-Hicks contractions.
B. Premature onset of labor.
C. An obstetrical emergency.
D. Both A and B.

7. What is the average length of labor for a woman having her first baby (primigravida)?

A. 4 hours.
B. 8 hours.
C. 15 hours.
D. 24 hours.

8. In a normal pregnancy, a mass palpated midway between the umbilicus and symphysis pubis indicates about which month of pregnancy?

A. Second month.
B. Fourth month.
C. Seventh month.
D. Ninth month.

9. You are called to the home of a woman experiencing vaginal bleeding with no history of trauma. How can you best evaluate her condition?

A. Ask her husband how much she has been bleeding.
B. Take postural vital signs.
C. Ask her how many pads she used per hour during a normal menstrual period.
D. Check the pad she has in place for the amount of blood present.

10. Select the most appropriate statement regarding the care of a rape patient.

    A. The patient should be allowed to bathe prior to transportation to the hospital.
    B. When taking patient history, it is important for the paramedic to collect evidence as well as solicit medical history.
    C. The genitalia should always be examined for injury prior to transport.
    D. The paramedic should limit the physical exam and should care for only those injuries requiring immediate stabilization.

11. Select those statements that are true:

    (1) An incomplete AB exists when the fetus died at less than 20 weeks and is retained in the uterus for at least two months.
    (2) An inevitable AB is one in which all products of conception have not yet been passed vaginally.
    (3) A missed AB is characterized by vaginal bleeding during pregnancy and softening of the cervix.
    (4) A spontaneous AB occurs naturally and may be mistaken for heavy menstrual flow.
    (5) A threatened AB is a situation in which there is slight cervical dilatation and the fetus remains alive.

    A. 1, 2, 4.
    B. 1, 3, 5.
    C. 2, 4, 5.
    D. 2, 3, 4.

12. During pregnancy, total maternal blood volume is increased by:

    A. 30%.
    B. 60%.
    C. 90%.
    D. 120%.

13. The frequency of contractions is measured from the time of the:

    A. Beginning of one contraction to the beginning of the next contraction.
    B. Beginning of one contraction to the end of the same contraction.

C. End of one contraction to the beginning of the next contraction.

D. Onset of pain until the pain has subsided.

14. Your patient has sustained perineal lacerations during childbirth. You should include all of the following in the prehospital care of this patient *except*:

A. Pack the vaginal os with sterile gauze.

B. Application of direct pressure.

C. Have the patient hold her legs together.

D. Administer high-concentration oxygen.

15. Your patient is a 38-year-old who is approximately seven months pregnant and presents with a chief complaint of vaginal bleeding. She denies abdominal pain or cramping. You would suspect this patient's problem is due to:

A. Ruptured ectopic pregnancy.

B. Abruptio placenta.

C. Uterine rupture.

D. Placenta previa.

16. You are called to a shopping mall to care for a 17-year-old patient who states she is 8 months pregnant. She complains of dizziness and severe headache. Vital signs are pulse 80, respirations 14, BP 162/98. Her rings appear to be impairing her circulation, and you offer to take them off. As you are assisting her, she becomes unresponsive and exhibits tonic-clonic movements. You suspect:

A. Eclampsia.

B. Idiopathic epilepsy.

C. Pregnancy-induced hypertension.

D. Supine hypertensive syndrome.

17. Which of the following could be included in the prehospital care for the preceding patient?

A. Apply PASG.

B. Administer diazepam 5–10 mg IV.

C. Start an IV with normal saline.

D. Transport rapidly with lights and sirens.

18. You are dispatched on a possible OB case. Upon arrival, you find a 29-year-old female who is gravida 6, para 3, AB 0 with an expected date of confinement (EDC) 10 weeks from this date. She complains of a constant tearing pain in her abdomen, nausea, and slight vaginal bleeding. Her pulse is 120, respirations 22/shallow, BP 100/60. You would suspect:

A. Placenta previa.
B. Placenta abruptio.
C. Amniotic embolism.
D. Uterine rupture.

19. What is the appropriate dose of oxytocin that is added to an IV solution?

A. 0.5 units.
B. 5 units.
C. 20 units.
D. 50 units.

20. You have found it necessary to complete a delivery at the scene. When the baby's head emerges, you notice that the cord is wrapped tightly around the neck twice. You would:

A. Quickly place two umbilical clamps and cut between them.
B. Immediately begin transportation to the closest hospital.
C. Gently loosen the cord and pull it over the baby's head.
D. Carefully push the head upward and transport the patient.

21. You have been called by the sister of a 38-year-old who is in active labor. She is a gravida 5, para 3, with contractions two minutes apart. The sister is insisting that you transport her to the hospital immediately. Which of the following factors is *least* important to your decision regarding transport?

A. The patient's age.
B. History of five pregnancies.
C. Contractions two minutes apart.
D. The patient's urge to push.

22. If difficulties arise during the delivery of a neonate's upper shoulder, you can facilitate delivery by gently:

A. Pulling on the shoulders.
B. Guiding the head upward.

C. Guiding the head downward.
D. Pushing the head backward.

23. When the head of the baby begins to push out of the vagina during a contraction, you should:

   A. Encourage the woman to breathe deeply and slowly.
   B. Gently pull the vagina open from both sides to allow passage of the baby.
   C. Apply gentle pressure to the baby's head, using the palm of your hand.
   D. Slide your finger past the baby's head and check for the possibility of the umbilical cord around the baby's neck.

24. You find it necessary to complete delivery of a 25-year-old multipara at home. As the baby's head emerges, you note that the membranes remain intact. Management of this situation requires you to:

   A. Support the baby's head and transport in this position STAT.
   B. Use a scalpel to peel the membranes as the baby emerges.
   C. Remove the cord from the baby's neck without disturbing the membranes.
   D. Puncture the membranes as soon as the head is delivered and remove from the baby's face.

25. You have delivered an infant whose mother admits to using heroin during the latter stages of labor. What is the neonatal dosage of the drug indicated in this situation?

   A. 0.02 mg/kg.
   B. 0.1 mg/kg.
   C. 0.3 mg/kg.
   D. 0.5 mg/kg.

26. Delivery of the placenta generally occurs how many minutes following birth of the baby?

   A. 2–3.
   B. 5–10.
   C. 20–30.
   D. 60.

27. During the resuscitation of a newborn, you have found it necessary to provide positive-pressure ventilation. Which of the following statements applies to the bag-valve device necessary in this situation?

    A. The bag volume should be >750 ml.
    B. The pop-off valve must be bypassed.
    C. A large bag is necessary to provide adequate tidal volumes.
    D. An anesthesia bag is best because it requires less training.

28. You note thick, green particulate matter in the amniotic fluid during delivery. Management in this situation requires you to:

    A. Vigorously stimulate respiratory effort.
    B. Assemble endotracheal intubation equipment.
    C. Minimize efforts that induce respirations.
    D. Both B and C.

29. What is the preferred vascular access route during the resuscitation of the neonate?

    A. Brachiocephalic.
    B. Umbilical vein.
    C. Basilic vein.
    D. Cephalic vein.

30. You perform a field delivery without difficulty. On evaluation for the initial Apgar score, you note the following: The body is pink and extremities are blue; pulse rate is 80; infant grimaces and cries when stimulated and moves actively with a good strong cry. What is the baby's Apgar score?

    A. 6.
    B. 7.
    C. 8.
    D. 9.

31. The neonatal dosage of epinephrine 1:10,000 is:

    A. 0.01–0.03 ml/kg.
    B. 0.03–0.05 ml/kg.
    C. 0.1–0.3 ml/kg.
    D. 1.0–3.0 ml/kg.

32. Positive-pressure ventilation is indicated for a neonate in all of the following situations *except*:

    A. Heart rate <100 per minute.

    B. Acrocyanosis persisting after supplemental oxygen.

    C. Respiratory rate 40 to 60 per minute.

    D. Apnea that does not respond to stimulation.

33. A few moments following birth, a neonate becomes unresponsive, apneic, and pulseless. Which of the following statements is correct regarding CPR in this situation?

    A. Both thumbs are positioned on the middle third of the sternum; compression depth is 1/2 to 3/4 inches; rate is 120/min.

    B. The index and middle fingers of one hand are placed on the intermammary line; compressions are 1/2 to 3/4 inches; rate is at least 100/min.

    C. The index finger is placed one finger-breadth below the intermammary line; compression depth is 1/4 to 1/2 inches; rate is 80–100/min.

    D. Either A or B is acceptable.

34. You have just completed delivery of a baby in the home. After you cut the cord, the proud father wants to hold his son while you prepare his wife for transport to the hospital. What risk do you anticipate in this situation?

    A. The father might drop the baby and blame your crew.

    B. The baby could develop respiratory distress without warning signs.

    C. The father may become agitated and report you to the Medical Director if you do not cooperate.

    D. The baby is vulnerable to hypothermia and requires immediate care.

35. Which of the following is *not* an acceptable source of warming for the infant during neonatal transport?

    A. Chemical heat packs.

    B. Hot water bottles.

    C. Rubber gloves filled with warm water.

    D. Radiant-heating units.

36. What are the initial steps in neonatal resuscitation (in order)?

    A. Positioning, ventilation, suctioning, tactile stimulation.

    B. Positioning, suctioning, tactile stimulation, ventilation.

    C. Ventilation, tactile stimulation, suctioning.

    D. Tactile stimulation, positioning, ventilation.

Answers with Rationale

1. (B) The placenta functions as a transfer mechanism for oxygen, nutrients, and antibodies. It also stores nutrients and excretes CO_2 and waste materials. Hormones that maintain pregnancy are produced by the ovaries.

2. (D) Pelvic inflammatory disease (PID) is an acute or chronic infection that may involve the uterus, ovaries, fallopian tubes, and adjacent structures. Causative organisms include gonorrhea (most common), staphylococcus, streptococcus, and chlamydia as well as other microorganisms. If untreated, it can result in the need for complete removal of the reproductive organs or generalized sepsis. Renal calculus (kidney stone) does not produce bilateral lower quadrant pain and tenderness. Amenorrhea is defined as the absence of menstruation. BSO is an abbreviation for bilateral salpingo-oophorectomy, the surgical removal of both fallopian tubes and ovaries.

3. (A) Fertilization of the ovum, or egg, that is produced by the ovaries normally occurs in the fallopian tubes. The egg travels through the fallopian tubes with the help of cilia. The endometrium is the internal lining of the uterus that provides nourishment to the fertilized egg. If fertilization does not occur, the endometrium—composed of cells and blood—is shed by the uterus during the menstrual period (about once a month). The vagina is the muscular tube that connects the uterus to the external genitalia.

4. (C) Labor is divided into three stages. The first stage of labor begins with contractions and ends with cervical dilatation. The second stage then begins and ends with the baby's birth. This also marks the beginning of the third stage, which ends with placental delivery. Prehospital administration of oxytocin (Pitocin) should never precede neonatal delivery due to complications (e.g., explosive delivery, uterine rupture, neonatal hypoxia, etc.).

5. (B) Ectopic pregnancy occurs when a fertilized ovum implants anywhere other than the uterine cavity, most commonly in the fallopian tube (95% of all ectopics). Most ruptures occur before the woman suspects she is pregnant or shortly after pregnancy is confirmed. Last normal menstrual period (LMP) is usually between 6–8 weeks prior to the onset of

symptoms and is commonly associated with intermittent spotting. Referred shoulder pain is present in 15–20% of cases. PID is usually associated with a purulent, heavy vaginal discharge. Dysmenorrhea is defined as painful menstruation. Salpingitis, or inflammation of the fallopian tubes, does not cause referred shoulder pain.

6. (A) Braxton-Hicks contractions, or false labor, begin during the early weeks of pregnancy and occur throughout. Early episodes cause no discomfort for the patient and usually go unnoticed. As she nears term, these contractions may cause discomfort due to increased uterine size. They are characteristically irregular and ease with walking, whereas true contractions are regular and intensify with walking. No intervention is necessary.

7. (C) The average length of labor for a primigravida is 15 hours. (Multigravida means multiple pregnancies.) When assessing a mother to determine if delivery is imminent, you should ask if it's her first baby, how long she has been in labor, frequency and duration of contractions, if she has an urge to move her bowels, and if she is under a doctor's care. Finally, you should examine for crowning if the history gathered leads you to believe delivery is imminent. Explain the process to the patient and respect her privacy.

8. (B) The fundus (top of uterus) is usually located between the umbilicus and symphysis pubis during the fourth month of pregnancy. Before the fourth month, the fundus is not easily palpated. At the fifth month, it is usually at the umbilicus. Discovery of the fundus, or perhaps a mass, in an unexpected location during a given time may indicate a complication.

9. (B) When you are examining a woman who has vaginal bleeding, you can determine if blood loss is significant by checking her pulse rate in both the sitting and supine positions. If, when moved from supine to sitting, the pulse rate increases by 20 beats or more per minute, or if the blood pressure drops by 15 mm Hg or more, she probably has lost at least one unit of blood. She should be treated for impending shock.

10. (D) When caring for a rape patient, it is important for you to limit the physical exam and care of the patient to only those injuries that require immediate stabilization. It is important that you protect the patient's privacy and feelings. Physical evidence may be lost if the rape victim is allowed to bathe. The genitalia should be examined only if obvious

bleeding must be controlled. Keep in mind that your primary mission is patient care. Do not cut or tear clothing from the patient, since valuable evidence may be disrupted. Law enforcement personnel will gather and protect evidence. Your report form must be very complete.

11. (C) Incomplete abortion (AB) is one in which some but not all products of conception have been passed vaginally. A missed AB is one in which the fetus died in utero and is retained. Although there is no vaginal bleeding associated with missed AB, serious infection results from nonviable, retained products of conception.

12. (A) Increased blood volume of at least 30% is necessary to maintain placental circulation, which provides the developing fetus with nutrition and oxygen. Additional maternal demands coincide with this increase including increased cardiac workload, vascular pressure and metabolism. It is important to remember the additional circulating blood volume in management of a traumatized pregnant patient because customary signs of hypovolemia will not develop as quickly as normally expected.

13. (A) Determining the frequency of contractions is important in the assessment of a patient in labor. They are timed from the beginning of one contraction to the beginning of the next contraction. Duration is determined from the beginning of a contraction, when the uterus begins to tighten, until the end of the same contraction, when the uterus becomes soft. Pain is not reliable because there is an interval at the beginning of the contraction during which the patient does not experience discomfort.

14. (A) You should never pack the vaginal opening, or os, with anything due to the extreme risk of contamination. Application of direct pressure can be accomplished by manually holding a perineal pad or sterile multiple trauma dressing in place or by placing it between the patient's legs and instructing her to hold her legs tightly together. The decision is based largely on the location of the lacerations and the patient's ability to cooperate. Any patient who is bleeding should receive oxygen therapy.

15. (D) Placenta previa results from placental implantation in the lower uterine segment. It may partially or completely cover the internal cervical os. Bleeding usually begins in the third trimester as the cervix begins to thin, or efface. Placenta previa is associated with painless, massive external hemorrhage. Predisposing factors for previa include multiparity, rapid succession of pregnancies, and maternal age >35 years.

16. (A) The patient initially presented with pregnancy-induced hypertension (PIH). PIH is the obstetrical term used more commonly than preeclampsia. Once the seizure activity occurred, her diagnosis became eclampsia. Signs and symptoms of PIH include hypertension, edema, headache, epigastric pain, and blurred vision. Idiopathic epilepsy is seizure disorder of unknown cause. While the patient could be epileptic, the presenting signs and symptoms are consistent with PIH and eclampsia. Supine hypertensive syndrome does not exist.

17. (B) Management of a patient with eclamptic seizures in the field includes diazepam 5–10 mg slow IV push. Management also includes maintenance of the airway, providing oxygen, and administration of magnesium sulfate 2–4 g IV of 10% solution, if available. Normal saline is contraindicated due to the sodium content. Since the patient is hypertensive, PASG is not indicated. She should be transported quietly, in a left lateral position, in a darkened environment, if possible, to avoid sensory stimulation.

18. (D) Uterine rupture is characterized by sudden, severe abdominal pain generally described as "ripping or tearing." Although external bleeding may be either minimal or absent, profound shock results from internal hemorrhage. Placenta previa presents with painless, massive external hemorrhage. Premature separation of a normally implanted placenta is known as placenta abruptio. Severe abdominal pain and uterine rigidity are associated with an abruption. Prehospital differentiation of a ruptured uterus from placenta abruptio may be accomplished by palpating the location of the fundus (top of the uterus). The fundus is usually felt below the umbilicus when the uterus has ruptured. Amniotic embolism affects the mother and can occur after the baby has been born. Signs and symptoms include sudden tachypnea, tachycardia, and/or hypotension.

19. (C) Oxytocin is a naturally occurring hormone that increases electrical and contractile activity in uterine smooth muscle. It can initiate or enhance rhythmic contractions at any time during pregnancy. It has a rapid onset of action and a very short half-life. Prehospital administration of oxytocin (Pitocin) may be indicated to control postpartum uterine bleeding after placental delivery when uterine massage is ineffective or the patient develops hypovolemic shock. You must determine that there is not another undelivered fetus. Oxytocin may be administered IV or IM. The IV dose is 10–20 USP units (20 mg per 10 USP units) in

1000 ml of a crystalloid solution at 20–30 macrodrops/minute titrated to severity of hemorrhage and uterine response. If you are unable to start an IV, 10 USP units may be administered IM. Lactated Ringer's or D_5/LR is IV fluid of choice. Oxytocin administered with D_5W may result in water intoxication due to the required volume and rapid metabolism of the dextrose in this solution.

20. (A) If the umbilical cord is wrapped tightly around the neonate's neck, you must place two clamps on the cord, cut between them, and deliver the baby as quickly as possible. Once the umbilical cord has been severed, the baby is without life support. If transport was started immediately, delivery would continue with subsequent pulling or tearing of the cord. Attempting to loosen a cord which is wrapped twice tightly around the neck will delay management. Pushing the baby's head upward may result in cord compression or laceration. Tension on the cord causes neonatal anoxia. Critical neonatal blood loss as well as anoxia result from a torn cord.

21. (A) The patient's age is not as important as the history of multiple pregnancies, the contraction intervals, and the patient's urge to push. Delivery in the multipara usually proceeds rapidly.

22. (C) Assisting delivery of the shoulders is not uncommon or difficult. Generally the upper shoulder delivers first. Gently guiding the baby's head downward allows the shoulder to slide under the mother's symphysis pubis, or pubic bone. After the upper shoulder is delivered, the reverse maneuver is often needed for the lower shoulder.

23. (C) As the baby's head begins to push out of the vagina, gently press against the head with the palm of your hand, preventing an explosive birth. Avoid pushing in on the soft areas (fontanelles) of the baby's head, as the brain is just below the skin. Encourage the patient to pant during contractions to relieve some of the urge to push. You should avoid touching the vagina and can check for her presence of the cord around the baby's neck after the head is delivered.

24. (D) Immediate rupture of the amniotic sac is indicated upon discovery. Use a clamp to perforate the sac. Clear the sac from the baby's nose and mouth as soon as the head is delivered. Suction thoroughly to prevent aspiration of amniotic fluid.

25. (B) Narcan (naloxone) is an effective narcotic antagonist. Heroin is a drug that crosses the placental barrier. Since the mother admitted using the drug shortly before delivery, you must anticipate a depressed neonate. Respiratory depression is managed by rapidly administering IV naloxone 0.1 mg/kg of a 0.4 or 1.0 mg/ml solution. The initial dose may be repeated every 2–3 minutes as needed. Since naloxone may precipitate acute withdrawal, caution must be used when administering it to a neonate of a narcotic-addicted mother. Naloxone may be given ET, IM, or SQ if an IV cannot be established.

26. (C) Placental delivery generally takes 20–30 minutes in either a primigravida or multigravida patient. This is useful for the paramedic to know since a decision must be made after a field delivery whether or not to delay transport until after delivery of the placenta. Uterine massage should be instituted once the placenta separates from the uterus.

27. (B) Most bag-valve devices have a pressure-limited pop-off valve that vents the compressed volume outside when the pressure exceeds 30–35 cm of water. This valve must be closed because the neonate's initial breaths may require higher pressure in order to inflate its unexpanded lungs. Bag volume should be ≤750 ml because larger bag volumes do not accurately provide for an infant's small tidal volume. Use of the anesthesia bag requires more training and skill than does a bag-valve device due to the exceptionally high pressures which it can deliver.

28. (D) Meconium is a dark-green thick material found in the intestine of the neonate. Normally it is expelled a few hours following birth. If passed in utero, it usually indicates fetal distress. This may be due to placental insufficiency or cord compression, resulting in hypoxia. Severe pulmonary inflammation, reversion to fetal circulation, and atelectasis result from meconium aspiration. If the meconium is thin, it can be adequately removed with the bulb tip syringe as the head delivers. If the meconium is thick, efforts to induce spontaneous breathing must be minimized until the vocal cords are visualized. Tracheal suctioning is accomplished by application of a meconium aspirator directly to the endotracheal tube. The baby is then intubated, suctioned, intubated, suctioned, and so on until the meconium has been removed. After these efforts, respiratory stimulation is applied and 100% oxygen administered. Meconium aspiration is one of the leading causes of neonatal mortality.

29. (B) The preferred vascular access site for a neonate is the umbilical vein because it is easily recognized and cannulated. The umbilical cord has three vessels—two arteries and one vein. After the umbilical cord is cut, the arteries rapidly constrict, making the vein even more apparent. If needed, access is accomplished by trimming the umbilical cord to 1 cm above the abdomen with a scalpel. This procedure is not painful for the infant since the cord has no nerve innervation. A #5 French umbilical catheter is then inserted until a flow of blood is obtained. It is important not to insert the catheter too far because the liver is within a short distance of the umbilical vein. A three-way stopcock is applied, and fluid administration (lactated Ringer's or normal saline) is initiated very slowly, using microdrop tubing.

30. (C) An Apgar score of 10 is the highest score possible. This baby's score of 8 was determined as follows: appearance = 1, pulse rate = 1, grimace = 2, activity = 2, respirations = 2.

31. (C) Although medications are seldom necessary for neonatal resuscitation, epinephrine may used indicated to treat bradycardia (rate <80/minute) which is refractory to stimulation, warming, oxygenation, and ventilation. When needed, epinephrine 1:10,000 is administered at 0.1 to 0.3 ml/kg. It may be delivered endotracheally or intravenously.

32. (B) Acrocyanosis is cyanosis of the newborn's palms and feet. This is a common finding that persists for the first few hours of life. As peripheral circulation and thermoregulation are achieved, the discoloration disappears. If, however, central cyanosis persists after supplemental oxygen is administered, positive-pressure ventilation with an anesthesia bag is indicated.

33. (A) Chest compressions can be accomplished by encircling the baby's chest and placing both thumbs on the middle third of the sternum. Compressions are correctly performed from 1/2 to 3/4 inches at a rate of 120/minute. In the case of a large newborn, the two-finger method of infant CPR can also be used, at a rate of 120/minute. Assisted ventilation must always accompany chest compressions.

34. (D) Hypothermia is a major, immediate health risk for the newborn. After leaving an environment of at least 99.6°F, the wet baby is ushered into one that is usually much cooler. Body heat is lost at a much greater

rate through evaporation when the skin is wet. Heat loss also occurs by convection, radiation, and respirations. The development of hypothermia is facilitated by an infant's immature heat-regulating mechanism.

35. (A) Chemical heat packs should never be used for infant warming since the temperature of these packs can reach 50–60°C (122–140°F) and may cause severe burns. Hot water bottles and rubber gloves filled with warm water may be used, but the infant must be protected by several layers of blanket material. Radiant-heating units are available and may be very beneficial in maintaining body temperature.

36. (B) The newborn should be placed on his back with the neck slightly extended. Next, the mouth and then the nose should be suctioned. Additional tactile stimulation, such as gently slapping the soles of the feet or rubbing the infant's back, may be needed to induce respirations. Ventilation is then appropriate after these first steps.

7

Behavioral Emergencies

1. Which of the following is *not* a characteristic of an emotional crisis?

    A. A crisis is sudden.
    B. Normal coping mechanisms fail.
    C. A crisis typically lasts weeks to months.
    D. Emotional crisis can produce self-destructive or socially unacceptable behavior.

2. Which of the following approaches facilitates a therapeutic interaction with the patient in a crisis situation?

    A. Conveying authority, active listening, and focus on issues relating to the crisis.
    B. Reassuring the patient that he or she will be all right.
    C. Expressing concern toward the problems that underlie the crisis.
    D. Providing reassurance through the offer of possible solutions to the problems that led to the crisis.

3. Which of the following is *not* an objective of crisis intervention?

    A. Shield the victim from additional stress.
    B. Assist the victim in mobilizing his or her resources.
    C. Return the victim, as much as possible, to a precrisis level of functioning.
    D. Establish long-term goals for the victim.

4. What is the best approach to management of emotionally disturbed patients?

    A. Restrain them preventively.
    B. Avoid physical gestures of comfort initially.
    C. Administer sedation, such as Valium.
    D. Use touch to help calm them.

5. Which of the following statements is most correct regarding family, friends, and bystanders at the scene of a medical emergency?

    A. They can nearly always be helpful in calming an agitated patient.
    B. They should be ignored because the patient is the only one who requires your attention.

    C. They should be observed for extreme anxiety reactions, in response to the patient's condition, which might require your care.

    D. They should be asked to leave the patient area.

6. What are the important qualities and attributes for the paramedic to possess or develop, in order to deal effectively with behavioral emergencies?

    (1) Genuineness and sensitivity.

    (2) Extensive knowledge of psychology.

    (3) Ability to remain objective and nondefensive in response to patient behavior.

    (4) Ability to cope effectively with own emotional responses.

    A. 1, 2, 3.

    B. 1, 2, 4.

    C. 1, 3, 4.

    D. 2, 3, 4.

7. Which of the following statements is most correct regarding the patient history in the field for an individual with a behavioral emergency?

    A. It should be the same as a history in other patients.

    B. It should include information related to the behavioral problem and life situation.

    C. It should include only information about the behavioral problem.

    D. It is not needed in the field setting.

8. Which of the following are the most important first indicators of the patient's mental status?

    A. General appearance, mood, and level of consciousness.

    B. Thought processes and thought content.

    C. Perception, memory, and judgment of past events.

    D. Psychological reactions to the current situation.

9. Which statement best describes suicide or a suicidal gesture?

    A. It is a sign of weakness.

    B. It is usually an impulsive act.

    C. It constitutes a major public health problem.

    D. Everyone is at equal risk of becoming suicidal.

10. Which risk factors should you consider when assessing suicide potential?

    (1) Age and sex.
    (2) Economic status.
    (3) History of depression.
    (4) Prior attempts.
    (5) Educational level.

    A. 1, 2, 5.
    B. 2, 4, 5.
    C. 1, 3, 4.
    D. 2, 3, 4.

11. When managing a patient who is exhibiting paranoid behavior, the paramedic's primary concern is that the paranoid patient is:

    A. Suspicious and unpredictable and may become aggressive.
    B. Excitable and needs neutral treatment.
    C. Demonstrating a sign of minor psychiatric illness.
    D. Exhibiting the need for a physical assessment.

12. You are interviewing a patient who is exhibiting paranoid behavior. According to his wife, he has become increasingly suspicious and distrustful over the past several days. Which of the following management strategies would be most therapeutic?

    A. Maintain a friendly but distant neutrality.
    B. Agree with his delusions.
    C. Provide warmth and reassurance regarding his condition.
    D. Take the wife into the next room to interview her.

13. You are assessing a 30-year-old female patient who is disoriented. Which of the following approaches is most appropriate?

    A. Ignore the patient's disorientation and proceed to care for physical needs.
    B. Restrain the patient to prevent problems.
    C. Attempt to keep the patient aware of the person, place, time, and current situation.
    D. Focus on transporting the patient to the nearest psychiatric facility.

14. You are called to see a 24-year-old male patient who appears to be having an acute dystonic reaction to his phenothiazine psychiatric drug therapy. Which of the following actions is appropriate management for this patient?

    A. Transport to a psychiatric hospital.
    B. Instruct the patient to delete the next dose.
    C. Request an order for diphenhydramine (Benadryl).
    D. Administer syrup of ipecac.

15. Which of the following approaches is most appropriate in managing Sally, a patient who is delusional and/or hallucinating?

    A. Do not agree with Sally, but recognize her belief in her delusion or hallucination.
    B. Try to convince Sally that her delusion or hallucination is not real and, therefore, not frightening.
    C. Ignore her references to the delusion or hallucination.
    D. Agree with Sally to win her cooperation.

16. Your patient is a 32-year-old male who was involved in a vehicular accident at moderate speed. He sustained multiple small lacerations and abrasions, and he has an open angulated fracture of his right tibia. The exam of his head, chest, and abdomen are negative. Initial and repeat vital signs are normal. He continues to express to you that he is badly injured and is dying. Repeated assessment shows that his physical condition is stable and unchanged. Your repeated reassurances have no effect. Which of the following best describes his reaction?

    A. Phobia.
    B. Delusion.
    C. Hallucination.
    D. Illusion.

17. Anger is a response frequently encountered in the emergent or urgent field setting. Which of the following are common causes of anger from patients, family members, and friends?

    (1) Fear.
    (2) Feelings of helplessness.
    (3) Denial.
    (4) Guilt.
    (5) Pain or discomfort.

    A. 1, 2, 5.
    B. 1, 3, 5.
    C. 1, 2, 4, 5.
    D. 1, 2, 3, 4, 5.

18. You respond to the home of a 15-year-old girl who has inflicted superficial lacerations on both wrists. You dress her wounds and are transporting her to the hospital. She cries for a few minutes and then stops. What response would be *least* helpful at this point?

    A. "You seem very sad."
    B. "Please don't cry anymore."
    C. "Have you ever tried to kill yourself before?"
    D. "What kinds of problems have you been having?"

19. Which of the following disorders could result in abnormal behavior?

    (1) Thyrotoxicosis.
    (2) Cushing's syndrome.
    (3) Epilepsy.
    (4) Reye's syndrome.
    (5) Multiple sclerosis.
    (6) Hypoglycemia.

    A. 3, 4, 6.
    B. 1, 2, 3, 6.
    C. 2, 3, 4, 6.
    D. 1, 2, 3, 4, 5, 6.

20. Patrick, a 45-year-old male, complains of a sense of impending disaster and feelings of hopelessness and helplessness. His wife tells you that he has lost interest in his hobbies and refuses to associate with any of their friends. You suspect this patient is suffering from:

    A. Schizophrenia.
    B. Depression.
    C. Delusions.
    D. Paranoia.

21. Your patient states, "I am going to kill myself." Your best response would be:

    A. "Things can't be that bad."
    B. "Why are you saying that?"
    C. "How do you plan to kill yourself?"
    D. "Just come to the hospital with me and everything will be fine."

22. Terry is a 19-year-old who, according to her mother, awoke this morning with paraplegia. There is no past history of trauma or underlying

medical problems. When you approach Terry to complete the physical assessment, you find her lying calmly in bed. She is alert and oriented. You suspect this patient:

A. Is experiencing a hysterical conversion reaction.
B. Is a typical hypochondriac with no medical problem.
C. Is suffering from a hysterical seizure disorder.
D. Has a manipulative personality type and is catatonic.

23. Jordan, a 14-year-old male, has just fallen from his bicycle. He has numerous jagged facial lacerations. A neighbor informs you that his parents are gone at the present time and will not be back for several hours. Which reaction would be consistent with this patient's age group?

A. Very concerned with his injuries and possible scars.
B. More concerned about his bike than his injuries.
C. Uncooperative and resistant to treatment.
D. Unconcerned about his accident.

24. You respond to the scene of a minor automobile accident. There are no apparent major injuries and you proceed to assess the victims in the first car. The mother was a passenger and was holding her 2-year-old son when another motorist struck them from behind at a slow speed. Which approach would you take in assessing the child?

A. Place the child on the stretcher.
B. Allow the mother to hold the child.
C. Have your partner hold the child.
D. Perform visual assessment only.

25. What is the *least* common reaction of victims in a disaster situation?

A. Panic.
B. Anger.
C. Denial.
D. Confusion.

26. While transporting an 89-year-old female from a nursing home to the hospital, she continuously asks for her mother and father. What is your most appropriate action?

A. Do not repeat yourself since she will not understand what you say.
B. Tell her that her mother is waiting at the hospital.
C. Avoid explanations since this will confuse her.
D. Orient the patient to person, place, and time repetitively.

27. You are dispatched to a local office building. The patient is a 29-year-old male who is under the treatment of a psychiatrist for an emotional disturbance manifested by uncontrollable rage. He became threatening and violent when told he was going to be dismissed by his boss. Upon arrival you find the patient in the office armed with a knife and threatening the boss. The office personnel inform you that the police have been contacted. You see the patient lunge at the boss. He misses and steps back to his original position. What should you do first?

    A. Restrain the patient.
    B. Talk the patient down.
    C. Take the knife away from the patient.
    D. Move everyone away from the immediate area.

28. When intervening in a crisis situation that involves a child, all of the following are principles the paramedic should employ *except*:

    A. Prevent the child from seeing things that will be upsetting.
    B. Monitor conversations that the child is subject to hear.
    C. Perform painful procedures quickly, without explanation.
    D. Allow the child to make choices when appropriate.

29. En route to the hospital, a patient begins to explain how voices are telling him to do bad things. To facilitate the patient's self-expression, you should say:

    A. "Go on."
    B. "I don't hear any voices."
    C. "There are no voices. You are having hallucinations."
    D. "Why do you think they are telling you to do bad things?"

30. You must restrain and transport a patient for her own protection. Which of the following principles of patient restraint is *not* correct?

    A. Always pad restraints so that the patient is not injured.
    B. Reasonable force should be used when applying physical restraints.
    C. Avoid undue explanations of what is being done at the time.
    D. Never agree to remove restraints in exchange for good behavior.

31. Which of the following statements is most true concerning the suicidal person?

    A. People who talk about suicide do not commit suicide.
    B. Suicidal people are ambivalent about living or dying.
    C. Once a person attempts suicide, he or she is suicidal forever.
    D. Individuals who attempt suicide are mentally ill.

Answers with Rationale

1. (C) Crises are by nature short in duration. Most last only 24–36 hours. In rare situations, a crisis may continue over several weeks.

2. (A) The most therapeutic interaction with patients in crisis is to help them orient to reality, so you want to focus on the issues relating to the crisis. The most realistic way to reassure the patient is to establish your authority (which will relieve the patient, temporarily, of the burden of responsibility) and to employ active listening. Do not promise things that may not happen. Therefore, do not tell the patient that things will be all right. They may not. Interest in the problems that underlie the present crisis is irrelevant. It is nontherapeutic to offer a solution(s) for the patient's problems.

3. (D) Crisis intervention is aimed at active and temporary intervention to deal with the immediate problem and the directly related behaviors. It is not concerned with developing long-term goals. The paramedic should shield the victim from additional stress, assist him or her in mobilizing resources (family, etc.), and return the victim, as much as possible, to a precrisis level of functioning.

4. (B) An extremely anxious patient may have distortions of perception and could misinterpret a comforting gesture. At the stage of severe anxiety, the patient responds with automatic, not reasonable, behavior. Therefore, it is best to gain the permission of emotionally disturbed patients before touching them.

5. (C) The paramedic, or a partner, should evaluate the status of the "significant others" at the scene and then make the appropriate decision regarding their capacity for helpfulness and their reactions to the situation. They may be helpful, may further agitate the patient, or may experience severe anxiety reactions themselves and require care. By ignoring the others who are involved, the paramedic might lose significant assistance or fail to avert further emergencies.

6. (C) Genuineness, sensitivity, the ability to remain objective and nondefensive, and the ability to cope effectively with one's own emotional responses are all very important. These qualities, coupled with the sincere use of active listening and empathic response, enable the paramedic to effectively manage the patient with a behavioral emergency.

An extensive knowledge of psychology is not required to provide optimal care in the prehospital setting.

7. (B) The history should include any significant physical information and as much information as possible that relates to the behavioral problem. It should also include the patient's life situation. This information can facilitate more effective interactions with the patient, presently and during continuing care.

8. (A) While all of these symptoms provide information regarding the patient's mental status and are useful in gaining an understanding of the patient's problem, the most important first indicators are physical appearance, mood, and level of consciousness.

9. (C) The number of suicides each year is so great (over 25,000) that suicide is now regarded as a major public health problem. Suicide is not a sign of weakness and is rarely impulsive. It is an indication of a seriously troubled person, who has had a long emotional struggle. Certain individuals have greater risk factors than others.

10. (C) The high-risk candidate is older, male, has a history of depression (the most common cause of suicide), and has often suffered a recent loss or diminished status. A history of previous attempts is associated with 50 to 80 percent of suicide victims, and the more violent, potentially lethal, or painful the previous attempt(s), the more at risk that individual is for a second attempt. These and other risk factors have been identified. Although they are predictive for groups, they do not always predict for the individual. While a greater number of females than males attempt suicide, males are more successful because they use more lethal methods. Eight out of ten suicide victims give warnings or messages that they are contemplating suicide, so it is important to listen for this or elicit expression of these feelings. Suicide is not directly related to economic status or educational level.

11. (A) The paramedic's primary concern is that this patient may become dangerous if he holds the attitude of "I'll get them before they get me." The patient must be evaluated for this potential. While the paranoid patient does not usually require restraints, in some situations restraints will be necessary. To avoid provoking a hostile response, use a neutral but somewhat distant manner, as you tactfully but firmly persuade him

to go to the hospital. Paranoid behavior may be the result of physiologic imbalance as well as manifestation of a psychiatric disorder, so a complete physical assessment should be made after admission.

12. (A) When dealing with the patient who is displaying paranoid behavior, you should maintain a friendly but neutral manner. The paranoid patient would be suspicious and upset by too much warmth and reassurance. Be honest with the patient, and do not agree with his delusions to placate him. This is one circumstance when you should not take the wife or other family members into another room or area to interview them. This will only make the patient more suspicious.

13. (C) You should attempt to orient the patient to the present and help her to understand what is happening to her before beginning the physical assessment. You should continue this effort during the evaluation and transport. This may require several repetitions of your identity and what you are doing. The patient should be restrained only if safety demands this intervention. While disorientation is most commonly experienced with dementia and Alzheimer's disease among the elderly, it can also result from head injury, from metabolic disorders such as diabetes, and from alcohol or other drug ingestion.

14. (C) An acute dystonic reaction can be very distressing to the patient and may require field intervention. The treatment of choice is diphenhydramine, 50–75 mg. Change in medication dosage must be determined by the physician. Syrup of ipecac is not indicated as phenothiazines have anti-emetic properties.

15. (A) The paramedic should tell Sally, the delusional and/or hallucinating patient, that he (the paramedic) is not experiencing these ideas or visions, but he does believe that she is experiencing them. Other approaches will not be particularly effective and will hinder the development of trust in the paramedic by the patient.

16. (B) A delusion is a false belief that cannot be changed by reasoning or demonstration of facts to the contrary. A phobia is an intense or illogical fear of specific objects or situations. A hallucination is a false perception of images and sensations as if they existed in reality. An illusion is a mistaken or distorted perception of an object.

17. (C) Fear, feelings of helplessness, pain or discomfort, and especially guilt, may all trigger the emotion of anger. Denial is not usually related to anger. It causes one to dismiss, ignore, or minimize a problem, symptoms, or event.

18. (B) Do not ask the patient to refrain from expressing herself through crying. It may be therapeutic for her, even though it makes you uncomfortable. Stating your observation that she seems sad may encourage her to share her feelings. Enquiring about a history of suicide attempts is also appropriate. Acknowledging that she has problems and asking her to share them may also encourage her to relate her story.

19. (D) Thyrotoxicosis results in the excessive secretion of thyroid hormone. The disturbances produced by this endocrine imbalance can result in delirium, schizophrenia, psychosis, and extreme anxiety. Cushing's syndrome affects the adrenal glands, causing elevation of the circulating adrenal cortisones. Manifestations can include delusions, thought disorders, extreme excitability, memory loss, delirium, hallucinations, and marked anxiety. The postictal state following epileptic seizure activity can be mistaken for withdrawn, bizarre behavior. Reye's syndrome develops following viral infections and affects children and adolescents. Extreme personality changes are often associated with early onset. Patients with multiple sclerosis may experience depression, severe mood swings, and personality changes that may result in inappropriate behavior. The visual and speech difficulties, as well as sensory losses associated with multiple sclerosis, parallel the manifestations of hysteria. Hypoglycemia may result in personality changes, restlessness, staggering gait, aggressiveness, and other symptoms commonly associated with substance abuse.

20. (B) Depressed individuals can be recognized by their melancholy appearance, listless or apathetic behavior, and loss of interest in others. They often express the desire to be isolated since they perceive that no one understands or cares about them. Schizophrenia is characterized by delusional thought processes and hallucinations. Delusions are false ideas or beliefs that represent a disturbance in the thought content and are indicative of a psychotic disorder. Delusions of persecution often lead to paranoia. Paranoid patients are suspicious and distrustful. Hostile and uncooperative, they provoke dislike and anger in those around them.

21. (C) Assessment of the patient's suicidal intent requires you to ask about the proposed method. The specificity of the plan and the lethality of the method are indicators of the patient's potential for self-destruction. Attempts to placate patients by indicating that you do not see their situation as "bad" will not establish a therapeutic relationship. "Why" questions should be avoided since they are intimidating. You must reinforce reality and must not make promises you cannot keep. Everything may not be "fine" if the patient goes to the hospital.

22. (A) The passive calmness that this patient is demonstrating toward her physical disability is indicative of a hysterical conversion reaction. Anxiety is reduced by converting her emotional state into a physical disorder. Hysterical conversion reactions produce physical symptoms that may mimic deafness, blindness, or paralysis and stem from strong emotional conflict. They may be very graphic in presentation and are seen in both men and women. It is beyond the scope of practice for the paramedic to differentiate between a conversion reaction and a physical disorder. Therefore, in the prehospital setting, the suspicion of hysterical conversion reaction should not alter serious attention to the management of the physical symptoms that prompted the call for emergency medical care.

23. (A) When you are managing pediatric patients during a period of crisis, it is important to remember the principles of growth and development as well as those of crisis intervention. The adolescent is particularly concerned with physical appearance. Preoccupation with physical appearance compounds the fear of deformity and permanent disability. You must be prepared to manage Jordan's anxiety over the lacerations, the separation from his parents, and the crisis situation itself.

24. (B) Toddlers have normal fears of interaction with strangers and separation from parents. It is important to allow the child to be with his mother during the physical examination. It is a challenge to assess this age group under any circumstance. You should not overwhelm the child by proceeding with "business as usual." Allowing the child to see what is being done and that no one is going to "ambush" him will facilitate the toe-to-head assessment. The reverse order of the secondary assessment will facilitate physical examination since the child will not perceive this activity as an attack.

25. (A) Panic is usually absent during most disasters. Only about ten percent of victims react with panic. Most react actively. During the various phases of the crisis, victims commonly experience anger, denial, and confusion.

26. (D) Elderly patients are prone to confusion for a number of reasons. Isolation, medications, fluid and electrolyte imbalances, and cardiovascular disease are but a few of the causes for mental lapses. It is important that prehospital professionals demonstrate respect for the patient through therapeutic interactions. If the patient is confused, using the patient's name will facilitate orientation. Terms of endearment (e.g., grandma, etc.) should be avoided since they are familiarities to which the paramedic is not entitled. Repetitive reinforcement of person, place, and time is beneficial in many situations.

27. (D) This patient is demonstrating homicidal tendencies during his rage. Restraining and disarming should be accomplished by the police, not by the paramedic. Concern for personal safety, as well as the safety of others, dictates that the first course of action is to clear the area. If the patient is paranoid as well as angry, removal of the bystanders will prevent him from perceiving their interest in the situation as threatening. Since the patient is out of control with his anger, there is no benefit in attempting to "talk him down."

28. (C) A child's trust is built on the truth. If a painful procedure must be performed, the paramedic should explain before it is done that the child will experience pain for a short period of time. It is important to tell the child that it is all right to cry. It is also important to demonstrate acceptance and empathy.

29. (A) The use of noncommittal words or phrases (e.g., "I see" or "Go on") or nonverbal communications (e.g., a nod of the head) are associated with the technique of facilitation. Facilitation can be used to return patients to previous topics when more information is required. If the patient asks you if you hear the voices, reality reinforcement requires an honest answer, "I don't hear any voices." Within the limited scope of prehospital crisis intervention, you should not make attempts to destroy the patient's reliance on the hallucinations. Since all behavior has meaning, it may require intense psychotherapy to identify the need that resulted in this behavior. "Why" questions should be avoided since they are intimidating.

30. (C) When applying restraints, you must always explain what you are doing, even when the patient does not appear to be listening. Restraining patients makes them feel as though they are losing even more control over the situation, compounding their sense of helplessness. If they perceive the restraint as a physical attack, they may respond with violent outbursts.

31. (B) Most suicidal people are ambivalent about living or dying. They often gamble with death, leaving others to save them. Eight out of ten people who kill themselves have given definite warnings, often verbal. People who wish to kill themselves usually hold this desire for a limited period of time, not forever. Although people who attempt suicide may be very distressed and/or depressed, they are not necessarily mentally ill.

8 Situational Review

You are dispatched to "an unconscious party." Upon arrival, you find a 61-year-old female, Mrs. Brink, lying on the kitchen floor. A neighbor informs you that she last saw Mrs. Brink getting the newspaper approximately three hours ago. The patient responds only to deep, painful stimuli. Her skin is pale, cool, and dry. You note no signs of trauma. Vital signs are P 40 and weak, R 22 and shallow, BP 40/palpation. Jugular veins are collapsed. Four empty pill bottles, found near Mrs. Brink, are labeled: Cardizem (30 mg, #30); Isordil (10 mg, #30); Coumadin (0.5 mg, #100); and Aldomet (250 mg, #100).

1. Which of the medications could be responsible for the patient's hypotension?

    (1) Cardizem.
    (2) Isordil.
    (3) Coumadin.
    (4) Aldomet.

    A. 2, 3.
    B. 3, 4.
    C. 1, 2, 4.
    D. 1, 2, 3, 4.

2. After connecting the ECG electrodes to Mrs. Brink, you note the following rhythm:

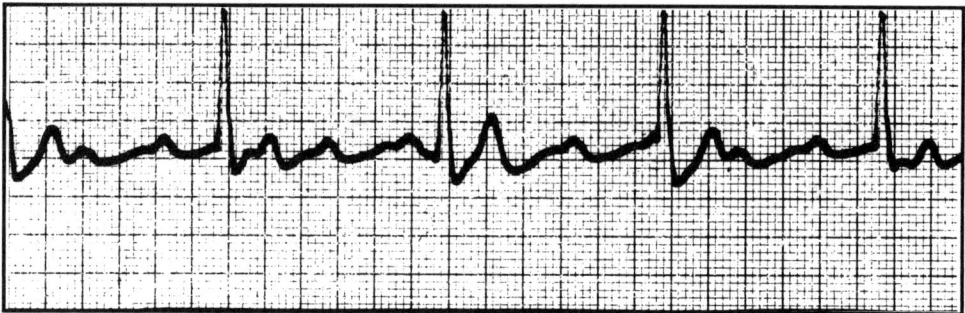

    You identify this dysrhythmia as:

    A. Third-degree AV block.
    B. Second-degree AV block, Type I.
    C. Second-degree AV block, Type II.
    D. Sinus bradycardia with high grade first-degree AV block.

3. Which medication is most likely responsible for this dysrhythmia?

   A. Aldomet.
   B. Isordil.
   C. Coumadin.
   D. Cardizem.

4. Which medications might be indicated in the treatment of Mrs. Brink?

   (1) Sodium nitroprusside.
   (2) Sodium bicarbonate.
   (3) Dopamine.
   (4) Atropine.

   A. 3, 4.
   B. 2, 3, 4.
   C. 1, 3, 4.
   D. 1, 2, 3, 4.

5. En route to the hospital with Mrs. Brink, you note the following ECG:

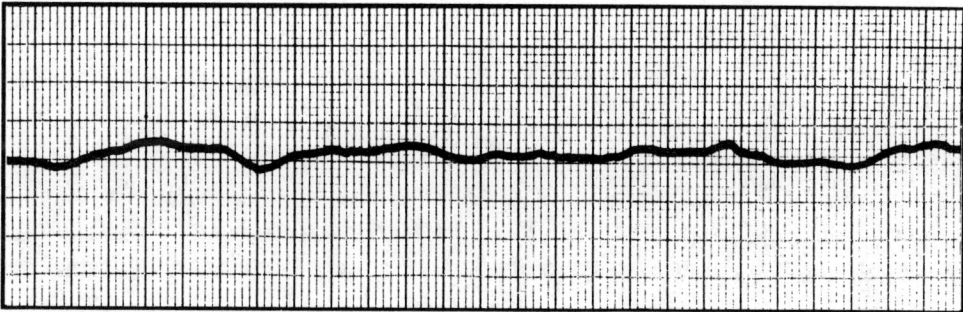

   You immediately:

   A. Deliver a precordial thump.
   B. Verify the rhythm in another lead.
   C. Administer atropine 1.0 mg IV push.
   D. Begin cardiopulmonary resuscitation.

You have been called to a football field where a 16-year-old boy has collapsed. He is unconscious and has the following vital signs: P 110, R 24, BP 90/60. His skin is cool and clammy. You note fine, generalized muscle tremors. There are what appear to be injection sites on both thighs. No one is able to give you any medical information regarding the patient's history.

6. Which of the following is the first priority in management of this patient?

   A. Strip test blood for glucose determination.
   B. Intravenous injection of naloxone.
   C. Dopamine drip IV to maintain the BP at 90 systolic.
   D. IV fluid challenge of 20 cc/kg.

7. After initial treatment has been rendered, the patient begins to make nonpurposeful responses to verbal stimuli. You would:

   A. Monitor the patient for 5 minutes before transport.
   B. Administer another IV dose of naloxone.
   C. Increase the IV fluid infusion rate.
   D. Administer a bolus of glucose, 25 grams.

8. What additional signs and/or symptoms would you suspect this patient might also exhibit as he begins to respond to treatment?

   (1) Hyperpnea.
   (2) Tachypnea.
   (3) Agitation.
   (4) Polydipsia.

   A. 2, 3.
   B. 3, 4.
   C. 1, 2, 4.
   D. 1, 2, 3, 4.

You are called to the scene of a "man down." On arrival, you find a 71-year-old male in cardiopulmonary arrest. No one knows how long the patient has been unconscious. The patient is pulseless and apneic. The pupils are dilated and react very sluggishly. CPR was started by a bystander prior to your arrival. The quick-look reveals the following ECG:

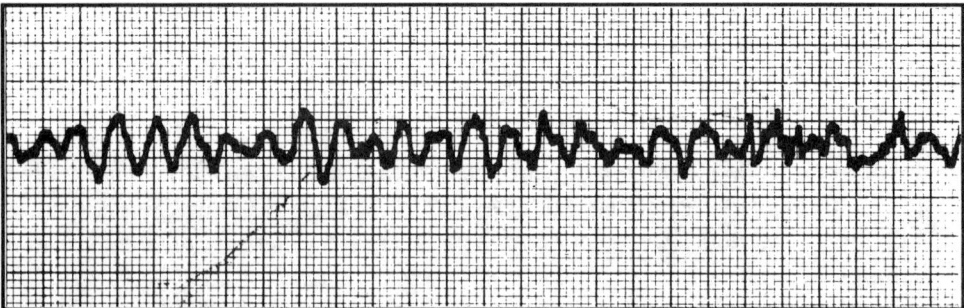

9. What is your first resuscitative measure?

   A. Defibrillate at 200–300 joules.
   B. Establish an IV of D$_5$W.
   C. Intubate the trachea and ventilate with 100% oxygen.
   D. Resume and continue CPR for at least two minutes.

10. The bystander suddenly stops CPR because the patient has vomited. What would you instruct the bystander to do?

    A. Pause for a moment to allow vomiting to stop and then resume CPR.
    B. Continue CPR with no interruptions to prevent brain damage from hypoxia.
    C. Stop CPR in order to prevent aspiration.
    D. Turn the victim to his side, apply the finger sweep, then reposition the patient, and resume CPR.

11. After intubating the trachea, ventilation is best accomplished with which of the following?

    A. Intermittent positive-pressure ventilator.
    B. Positive-negative pressure resuscitator.
    C. Resuscitator-inhalator.
    D. Bag-valve-mask device.

12. You are unable to establish a peripheral IV line. The base station physician has ordered an external jugular line. How would you approach this blood vessel when performing the venipuncture?

    A. At the apex of the triangle formed by the two heads of the sterno-mastoid muscle and the clavicle.
    B. Caudally and ventrally toward the suprasternal notch at an angle of 45° to the sagittal and horizontal planes.
    C. Midway between the angle of the jaw and the midclavicular line.
    D. Caudally toward the ipsilateral nipple and toward the junction of the middle and medial third of the clavicle.

You are called to an automobile accident with injury. The victim is a 19-year-old female, Eileen Ward. She was the passenger in a vehicle that was struck on the right front corner by a van. You notice the passenger's window has a starburst fracture, and Ms. Ward has minor bleeding from the right side of her head. She was not wearing a seat belt. Initially she was unresponsive and has now become combative and incoherent. Her vital signs are P 60, R 36 and shallow, BP 156/100. Her pupils are equal and react sluggishly. The remaining assessment is as follows: chest negative, abdomen guarded on palpation, and skin cool and dry. There is no significant external bleeding.

13. What is your initial assessment?

    A. Increased intracranial pressure secondary to a head injury.
    B. Neurogenic shock secondary to a spinal cord injury.
    C. Hypovolemic shock secondary to internal hemorrhage.
    D. Multiple trauma with possible drug and/or alcohol intoxication.

14. What IV fluid is indicated in the treatment of Ms. Ward?

    A. D_5W.
    B. Lactated Ringer's.
    C. 0.45 NaCl.
    D. 2% normal saline.

15. Which of the following infusion rates is most appropriate in this situation?

    A. 20 cc/kg.
    B. Sufficient to keep the vein open.
    C. 100 cc/hour.
    D. 150 cc/hour.

16. Given Ms. Ward's clinical presentation, which medication is initially indicated?

    A. 50% dextrose.
    B. Mannitol.
    C. Oxygen.
    D. Narcan.

You are dispatched to the home of Mrs. Winston. She is complaining of nausea and RUQ pain that began shortly after dinner. Assessment reveals a 40-year-old obese female in moderate distress. Her skin is warm and moist. Vital signs are as follows: P 106, R 24 and shallow, BP 140/92. Her abdomen is soft, with guarding noted in the RUQ. There is no history of similar episodes.

17. You suspect Mrs. Winston's problem is due to which of the following?

    A. Cholecystitis.
    B. Duodenal ulcer.

C. Renal calculi.
D. Pancreatitis.

18. Which of the following signs or symptoms is consistent with Mrs. Winston's medical problem?

A. Hemoptysis.
B. "Walking colic."
C. Acholic feces.
D. Hematemesis.

You are called to the scene of an automobile accident. The driver of the first car is unconscious, cool, and clammy. Auscultation of the chest reveals equal bilateral breath sounds and muffled heart sounds. Vital signs are P 140, R 36 and shallow, BP 80/70. Jugular veins are distended. There are no signs of injury other than a large ecchymotic area over the sternum.

19. What is the major life threat to this patient?

A. Flail chest.
B. Myocardial contusion.
C. Pericardial tamponade.
D. Tension pneumothorax.

20. Management of this patient includes all of the following *except*:

A. Rapid crystalloid IV infusion.
B. Rapid transport.
C. Endotracheal intubation.
D. Dopamine infusion.

The driver of the second car in the previous accident is slumped over the steering wheel. He is anxious and speaks in broken sentences. His skin is cool and clammy, P 124 and irregular, R 40 and shallow, BP 88/40. Asymmetrical and paradoxical chest wall movement is noted. Pupils are equal and reactive to light. No neurological deficits are noted.

21. Which of the following mechanisms accounts for the paradoxical chest wall movement on expiration?

A. Increased intrathoracic pressure.
B. Increased arterial oxygen tension.
C. Decreased intrathoracic pressure.
D. Decreased arterial oxygen tension.

22. Treatment for this patient includes:

    (1) Positive-pressure ventilation.
    (2) Securing the rib cage tightly with tape.
    (3) An IV solution of D_5W.
    (4) Bulky dressing taped to the bulging area.

    A. 1, 4.
    B. 2, 3.
    C. 1, 3, 4.
    D. 1, 2, 3, 4.

A female passenger in the second car is complaining of severe pain in the midshaft area of her left femur.

23. Immediate immobilization of this injury is important because the most acute complication of a fractured femur is:

    A. Hemorrhage.
    B. Fat embolism.
    C. Osteomyelitis.
    D. Avascular necrosis.

24. What is the best method of immobilizing the patient's leg?

    A. Air splint.
    B. Traction splint.
    C. Board splint.
    D. Posterior molded splint.

You are dispatched to the home of a patient with a medical problem. On arrival, you find a 23-year-old male with the chief complaint of vomiting and dizziness. He is pale, skin is clammy and slightly cyanotic. Lungs are clear on auscultation. You note ab-dominal tenderness on palpation. The patient admits to vomiting "coffee-ground" material for two days. Vital signs are P 140, R 30, and BP 96/64.

25. Which of the following would you suspect?

    (1) Hemorrhage due to esophageal varices.
    (2) Upper GI hemorrhage.
    (3) Lower GI hemorrhage.
    (4) Hypovolemic shock.

    A. 1, 4.
    B. 2, 4.

C. 3, 4.
D. 1, 2, 4.

26. How would you position the patient for transport?

   A. Trendelenburg position.
   B. Supine with legs elevated 45°.
   C. Semi-Fowler's position.
   D. Left lateral, head slightly lower than the feet.

27. Treatment for this patient may include high-flow O$_2$ and which of the following?

   A. IV of D$_5$W, dopamine drip.
   B. IV of lactated Ringer's, antishock garment.
   C. IV of lactated Ringer's, dopamine drip.
   D. IV of D$_5$W, antishock garment.

While off-duty and traveling alone, you stop at the scene of an automobile accident. You are met by a hysterical 35-year-old male screaming about the passengers, one of whom is his child. He is pointing to an automobile that is approximately 25 feet off the road down a 45° embankment. The vehicle has heavy damage to the front door on the passenger side.

28. Where would you expect to find the most badly injured patient?

   A. On the driver's side.
   B. On the passenger's side.
   C. In the back seat.
   D. Not enough information is known yet.

The automobile is a four-door sedan. You observe a 34-year-old female sitting in the front passenger seat. The door is caved in on her right leg. She is moaning about her right hip. In the back seat, lying behind the driver's seat, is a motionless female about 2 years old. Behind the passenger seat, sitting up very straight, is a 10-year-old female who is conscious but does not respond to your questions. She has noisy, labored respirations.

29. Select the proper order for examining the three patients in the car.

   A. 34-year-old, 10-year-old, 2-year-old.
   B. 2-year-old, 10-year-old, 34-year-old.
   C. 10-year-old, 34-year-old, 2-year-old.
   D. 10-year-old, 2-year-old, 34-year-old.

30. While initiating your assessment of the 2-year-old, you determine she is not breathing. Your first action is to:

    A. Start cardiac compressions.
    B. Give four quick breaths.
    C. Do nothing and move to the next patient.
    D. Open her airway.

31. The 10-year-old child has a flail section of the right lateral chest. Breath sounds on the right side are decreased, but the abdomen is soft. You note no obvious fractures of the long bones. Her vital signs are P 130, R 30, BP 80/P. What best defines flail chest?

    A. One rib fractured in two places.
    B. More than one rib fractured in more than one place.
    C. Three ribs fractured.
    D. Four ribs fractured.

You respond to a call from the husband of a 35-year-old female. The woman is 8 1/2 months pregnant and is experiencing bright red vaginal bleeding. She denies any pain.

32. Which of the following conditions is most likely?

    A. Ectopic pregnancy.
    B. Active labor.
    C. Ruptured uterus.
    D. Placenta previa.

33. Your patient's vital signs are P 90, R 16, BP 100/70. Which of the following actions is most appropriate?

    A. IV of D_5W and transport.
    B. Oxygen and transport.
    C. Oxygen, IV of D_5W, antishock garment inflated, and transport.
    D. Oxygen, IV of normal saline, antishock garment not inflated, and transport.

You are called to a scene where a 52-year-old male pedestrian was struck by a car traveling at a high rate of speed and was thrown approximately 100 feet. The patient was found lying on his side with a large laceration on the posterior scalp and an obvious open fracture of the left femur. The patient has snoring respirations at 12/min; breath sounds are difficult to assess due to the noisy environment. Other vital signs are P 115, BP 98/54.

34. What is your first priority in managing this patient?

    A. Provide a patent airway.
    B. Place the patient on a long spine board.
    C. Intubate.
    D. Control bleeding.

35. The patient responds to painful stimuli by extension and internal rotation of his arms and extension of his legs. This type of posturing is referred to as:

    A. Decorticate.
    B. Decerebrate.
    C. Flexion.
    D. Tetany.

36. Which sign would be *least* suggestive of increasing intracranial pressure in this patient?

    A. Hypotension.
    B. Bradycardia.
    C. Abnormal respiratory pattern.
    D. Pupil changes.

37. The patient's respirations are extremely noisy. When performing tracheal suctioning, how should the suction be applied?

    A. Only during insertion of the catheter.
    B. Only while removing the catheter.
    C. While the catheter is at the level of the carina.
    D. Both during insertion and removal of the catheter.

You are called to a private residence for a 61-year-old male patient complaining of heaviness in his chest that has persisted for one hour. The patient has a history of emphysema and "heart trouble." Medications include a "heart pill" and a "water pill." P is 52, R 24, BP 124/70. His ECG reveals a second-degree AV block, 2:1 conduction.

38. Despite the fact that you have been giving this patient oxygen at 4 L/min, he continues to become increasingly cyanotic. What should you do next?

    A. Intubate and ventilate with positive pressure.
    B. Give epinephrine to increase respiratory function.
    C. Reduce the oxygen flow rate.
    D. Increase the oxygen flow rate and be prepared to assist ventilations.

39. The patient then tells you that he takes large amounts of antacids for his "sour stomach." You might expect that he has developed:

    A. Respiratory alkalosis.
    B. Respiratory acidosis.
    C. Metabolic alkalosis.
    D. Metabolic acidosis.

40. You administer nitroglycerine to your patient. What is the usual dosage of nitroglycerine?

    A. 200 grains every 5 minutes, repeat three times.
    B. 0.4 mg, may repeat if needed.
    C. 5 mg initially, followed by 2 mg in 10 minutes.
    D. 0.5 grains, may repeat twice.

41. If the patient does not continue to tolerate this heart rhythm and rate, you anticipate administering atropine. Atropine is contraindicated in which condition?

    A. Glaucoma.
    B. Gout.
    C. Angina.
    D. Spastic colon.

You are called to the scene of a shooting. The victim is a 26-year-old male, approximately 180 lbs., in moderate distress. He is lying in a supine position on the floor. He is alert, oriented, and complaining of slight dyspnea. He is mildly cyanotic around the mouth and fingertips. His vital signs are P 100 and regular, R 24 and slightly shallow, BP 124/70. There are diminished breath sounds on the right side. There is a sucking chest wound with little bleeding at the level of the fifth intercostal space, anterior axillary line on the right side. This appears to be an entrance wound; there is no exit wound. Your assessment reveals no other apparent injuries.

42. What is your initial intervention?

    A. Place the patient on a cardiac monitor.
    B. Start an IV of lactated Ringer's or saline solution.
    C. Seal the wound with an occlusive dressing.
    D. Immobilize the thoracic spine.

43. After completing the assessment, you are concerned that the patient may develop a tension pneumothorax. You should be alert for which of the following signs indicating this condition may be occurring?

(1) Distended neck veins.
(2) Absence of breath sounds on affected side.
(3) Abdominal pain.
(4) Tracheal shift to the affected side.
(5) Signs of hypoxia.

A. 1, 2, 3.
B. 1, 3, 4.
C. 2, 4, 5.
D. 1, 2, 5.

44. During reassessment you observe that the patient is developing signs of a tension pneumothorax. Your initial intervention is to:

A. Open the occlusive dressing.
B. Perform a needle thoracostomy.
C. Perform a needle cricothyrotomy.
D. Insert an endotracheal tube.

45. If the previous intervention is unsuccessful, the next action is usually to:

A. Perform a needle thoracostomy.
B. Institute positive pressure ventilation.
C. Perform a needle cricothyrotomy.
D. Insert an endotracheal tube.

46. You are directed to perform a needle thoracostomy. The needle should be inserted at which location?

A. Second intercostal space, sternal border.
B. Fifth intercostal space, posterior axillary line.
C. Fifth intercostal space, sternal border.
D. Second intercostal space, midclavicular line.

47. Which of the following statements concerning spinal immobilization for this patient is most correct?

A. It is not necessary.
B. It is indicated if the patient complains of neck or back pain.
C. It cannot be done properly with a wound of this nature.
D. It should be performed with modifications for the injury.

Upon arrival at an industrial accident, you are informed that a large construction crane has tipped over, trapping Lincoln Jones beneath the rubble. You find Mr. Jones, a black male about 30 years old, with one leg pinned under the cab of the crane and the other leg, traumatically amputated, lying a short distance away.

48. Mr. Jones has a patent airway. You should next:

    A. Check for signs of shock by observing skin color in the axilla.
    B. Apply a tourniquet to the stump.
    C. Administer high-concentration O_2.
    D. Place saline dressings on the amputated lower leg.

49. Proper care for Mr. Jones' amputated lower leg includes:

    A. Placing it in an ice chest with dry ice.
    B. Soaking the limb in saline solution.
    C. Wrapping the limb in sterile aluminum foil and blankets.
    D. Wrapping the limb in a sterile burn sheet and placing it in a plastic bag in an ice chest.

50. Your patient has been extricated. He has a palpable but weak carotid pulse. You suspect a fractured pelvis and choose to apply an antishock garment. How would you apply the device?

    A. Inflate only the leg compartment encasing the still-attached leg.
    B. Inflate both leg compartments but not the abdominal compartment, as this may increase the blood loss from the stump.
    C. Inflate both leg compartments and the abdominal compartment.
    D. Apply a tourniquet to the stump, fill the area below the stump with ice packs, and then inflate all three compartments.

Answers with Rationale

1. (C) Although the mechanisms of action differ, Cardizem, Isordil, and Aldomet could all precipitate hypotension. As a calcium channel blocker, Cardizem decreases the availability of calcium resulting in an alteration of the magnitude and quantity of the excitation-contraction mechanism of the heart. It also decreases the contractility of the smooth muscle fibers of the blood vessels since these muscle fibers are also calcium dependent. Isordil is a form of nitrate and promotes vasodilation, as do all members of this drug family. The mechanism of action by which Aldomet lowers arterial pressure is not fully understood. Its beneficial action is thought to be due to its antiadrenergic actions (norepinephrine, epinephrine, and dopamine) at the tissue level. Coumadin is an anticoagulant and would not contribute to hypotension.

2. (A) The regularity of the P-P and R-R intervals and the lack of a relationship between the P waves and the QRS complexes indicates that the atria and ventricles are functioning independently of each other. This is the characteristic of third-degree, or complete, AV block.

3. (D) Cardizem is a calcium ion influx inhibitor, or slow channel blocker. Since this drug prolongs the refractory period of the AV node, it may cause abnormally slow heart rates and advanced degrees of AV block. Aldomet, in rare instances, may affect the SA node, resulting in sinus bradycardia. Isordil and Coumadin have not been reported to affect the heart rhythm.

4. (A) Dopamine is indicated in the treatment of hypotension resulting from the untoward effects of Cardizem, Aldomet, and Isordil. Atropine sulfate may be indicated in the treatment of advanced AV block due to Cardizem if there is no improvement in the blood pressure with dopamine therapy. Immediate transportation to the hospital is important since the patient might require a pacemaker if there is no clinical improvement with pharmacological intervention. Sodium bicarbonate would not be indicated without arterial blood gas reports. As a potent and rapidly acting vasodilator, sodium nitroprusside is effective in the management of heart failure and hypertension and, therefore, not indicated in this situation.

5. (B) Differentiating ventricular fibrillation and asystole is critical for selecting the appropriate treatment. In both cases, the patient is pulseless and apneic. In addition, ventricular fibrillation can masquerade as asystole on the ECG. Therefore, two different lead configurations should be checked to confirm the ECG diagnosis before initiating any of the resuscitative measures listed. It is important not to base the treatment of a patient solely on the information obtained from a machine. Always assess the patient first, then proceed to render care using the data obtained from diagnostic aids such as the ECG.

6. (A) Strip testing blood for glucose determination is indicated when treating an unconscious patient of unknown origin. If the reading is 45 mg/dl, or less, glucose 25 grams should be administered through a patent IV line. The injection sites on the thighs are typical locations for insulin administration. Naloxone is indicated in the treatment of an unconscious patient of unknown origin who does not respond to glucose and in the treatment of narcotic overdose. Dopamine should not be administered unless there is no improvement in the blood pressure after the initial treatment and until hypovolemia due to trauma has been ruled out. A fluid challenge is not indicated in the absence of a history of trauma.

7. (D) Due to a minimal response to the first bolus of glucose, it is important to administer a second bolus. The patient's blood glucose may have been so low that although there was slight improvement with one bolus, it was insufficient to raise the blood glucose enough to meet the metabolic needs of the brain.

8. (A) The response to the glucose is diagnostic of hypoglycemia. Additional signs and symptoms of hypoglycemia include agitation and tachypnea (rapid respirations) due to glucose deprivation of the central nervous system. Hyperpnea (unusually deep respirations) and polydipsia (excessive thirst) are signs consistent with hyperglycemia.

9. (A) The first resuscitative measure is to defibrillate the patient at 200–300 joules. If the initial defibrillation is unsuccessful, perform a second defibrillation. Transthoracic resistance is lowered by the first shock, resulting in more energy being delivered to the myocardium. If unsuccessful, administer a third shock at 360 joules. Resume CPR, intubate the trachea, and establish an IV line.

10. (D) The airway must be maintained at all times. If the patient vomits, the vomitus must be cleared from the oropharynx in order to prevent airway obstruction and aspiration. CPR is then resumed.

11. (D) The bag-valve-mask device is the most desirable for ventilating the patient because it conveys to the operator a sense of compliance of the lungs, indicating when more or less pressure is needed. This advantage is lost when an oxygen-powered device is used in the place of the bag. Due to the counter-pressure exerted during external chest compressions, the intermittent positive-pressure ventilator, positive-negative pressure resuscitator, and the resuscitator-inhalator prematurely stop the inspiratory cycle resulting in inadequate ventilations during CPR.

12. (C) The external jugular vein is approached midway between the angle of the jaw and the midclavicular line. The other three approaches are used when inserting an IV line into the internal jugular vein.

13. (A) The elevated blood pressure and borderline bradycardia are indicative of increasing intracranial pressure. As intracranial pressure increases, cerebral blood flow decreases, probably due to the mechanical effect of the pressure, causing a series of local compensatory changes in the cerebral vasculature. However, as the pressure continues to rise, these changes prove inadequate to maintain cerebral blood flow. The blood pressure begins to rise as a direct reflex effect of anoxia in the vasomotor area of the brain. The pulse slows as the blood pressure rises. The slowing pulse rate is one of the most reliable indications of increasing intracranial pressure. Neurogenic shock presents with hypotension and a normal pulse rate. Hypovolemic shock results in hypotension and tachycardia.

14. (B) Lactated Ringer's is the IV fluid of choice because it is an isotonic solution and remains in the vasculature. D_5W is not used because, although it is an isotonic solution, the dextrose moves into the cell within a short period of time, leaving hypotonic water in the vasculature. Both 0.45 NaCl and 2% normal saline are hypotonic solutions. When hypotonic solutions (e.g., 0.45 NaCl, 2% normal saline, and the remaining water from D_5W) are administered intravenously, osmosis causes the fluid to shift into the intracellular space in order to equilibrate the intravascular and intracellular concentrations. Therefore, these fluids may aggravate cerebral edema.

15. (B) The IV is used to maintain an open vein for drug administration, not fluid replacement in this situation. Rapid infusion of IV fluids aggravates cerebral edema and causes further increased intracranial pressure.

16. (C) The mainstay in treating the head-injured patient is the prevention of hypoxia and immediate hyperventilation with 100% oxygen. Following a head injury, there is an increase in the blood volume in the cranial cavity that is worsened by hypoxia, hypercarbia, and acidosis.

17. (A) The gallbladder is located in the right upper quadrant of the abdomen, and is responsible for storing bile until it is needed for fat digestion. The classical patient suffering from cholecystitis (inflammation of the gallbladder) is fair, fat, female, and forty. The pain associated with a duodenal ulcer is relieved by eating, whereas gallbladder pain occurs after eating when the inflamed gallbladder contracts in order to release bile into the small intestine. The pain associated with acute pancreatitis, although generally localized to the hypogastrium or to both upper quadrants, frequently penetrates straight through to the back. Renal calculi (kidney stones) produce pain that radiates from the abdomen or flank into the scrotum or labia.

18. (C) Acholic (absence of bile pigment) feces is a condition in which the stools become clay colored. This is due to an obstruction in the gallbladder that prevents bile from being released into the small intestine. In Mrs. Winston's case, this is most likely due to gallstones. Coughing up blood (hemoptysis) is associated with a pulmonary lesion. "Walking colic" is indicative of renal calculi. The patient is extremely restless and moves around in order to relieve the pain. In contrast, the patient with peritonitis is very still to prevent movement of an irritated peritoneal cavity. Hematemesis, vomiting blood, is caused by upper gastrointestinal bleeding.

19. (C) Jugular distention, narrowed pulse pressure, hypotension, and muffled heart sounds are signs of pericardial tamponade. When blood or fluid collects in the pericardial sac, mechanical compression of the heart results in increased venous and pericardial pressures and decreased arterial pressure. Muffled heart sounds result from the poor conduction of sound through fluid. Flail chest is suspected if asymmetrical chest wall movement and paradoxical respirations are present.

Sternal ecchymosis creates a high index of suspicion of myocardial contusion. However, this is not the immediate life threat and cannot be evaluated until the pericardial tamponade is corrected. Although the mediastinal shift associated with a tension pneumothorax causes increased venous pressure (jugular vein distention) and decreased arterial pressure due to the compression of the heart, breath sounds are not equal bilaterally. Breath sounds are absent on the affected side and diminished on the opposite side of the thorax. In the presence of a tension pneumothorax, the heart sounds are distant rather than muffled.

20. (D) Dopamine and other vasopressors are contraindicated in cases of hypovolemia. When hypovolemia is present, extreme degrees of vasoconstriction may occur and result in a critical decrease in organ blood flow even when a normal blood pressure is present. Crystalloid IV fluids (such as lactated Ringer's), endotracheal intubation, and rapid transport are indicated in the unconscious trauma patient in shock.

21. (A) During the expiratory phase of respiration, the intrathoracic pressure rises and is comparatively greater than atmospheric pressure. The increase in intrathoracic pressure causes outward bulging of the flail segment, giving rise to paradoxical chest wall movement. Conversely, during inspiration, the intrathoracic pressure falls below that of atmospheric pressure and results in inward collapse of the flail segment.

22. (A) Positive-pressure ventilation may reverse respiratory embarrassment. Utilize a bag-valve-mask and 100% oxygen. Taping a bulky dressing to the bulging area inhibits the outward excursion of a flail segment. Circumferential binding of the chest wall is contraindicated due to the resultant decreased ventilatory volumes. Dextrose IV solutions should not be utilized for volume replacement because the glucose enters the intracellular space, leaving hypotonic water in the vascular space.

23. (A) Significant blood loss can occur from a fractured femur and result in hypovolemic shock. Immobilization of the fracture and adequate fluid therapy may decrease the later complication of fat embolism. Osteomyelitis, or inflammation of the bone, is a complication of an open fracture when bacteria have entered the bone, particularly the marrow. This is also a later complication. Avascular necrosis of the femoral head is a complication of a hip dislocation that is not immediately reduced and stabilized.

24. (B) The best method for immobilizing a fractured femur is the traction splint. Reduction and immobilization of the fracture decreases further hemorrhage and injury and increases patient comfort by reducing painful muscle spasms. The air splint, with the exception of the pneumatic antishock garment, is not appropriate because it does not immobilize the fracture above and below the site of injury. A board splint, if properly applied laterally from the axilla to the foot, will suffice to immobilize the fracture when no other equipment is available. The posterior molded splint is a "half cast" and is applied to the posterior aspect of the entire leg to immobilize the extremity and does not apply traction.

25. (B) Blood from the upper gastrointestinal tract, which has been subjected to the gastric juices and digested, looks like old coffee grounds. The hypotension, tachycardia, and tachypnea are consistent with hypovolemic shock due to blood loss. Hemorrhage from ruptured esophageal varices is copious and usually bright red because it is not subjected to the digestive juices in the stomach. Lower gastrointestinal bleeding is characterized by melena, or black tarry stools.

26. (B) The physiological shock position is supine with the legs elevated. This position promotes venous return from the extremities without displacing the viscera against the diaphragm and interfering with respiration, which occurs with the Trendelenburg position (tilting the entire body so that the head is lower than the feet). Semi-Fowler's position is placing the patient in a sitting position with the head elevated approximately 45°. The left lateral position combined with the head below the level of the feet is indicated for patients with a venous air embolism. In this position, the the air embolus may be prevented from entering the pulmonary and arterial circulatory systems by "trapping" it in the right heart, preferably the right atrium.

27. (B) Lactated Ringer's and the pneumatic antishock garment may be indicated in the treatment of this patient due to hypovolemic shock. The use of the pneumatic antishock garment is currently controversial. Consult local protocols. Dextrose solutions are not used for fluid replacement because the dextrose does not remain in the vascular bed long enough to result in volume expansion. Dopamine and other vasopressors are contraindicated in the presence of hypovolemia.

28. (B) Since the vehicle has been hit on the right side, passengers seated on the right side of the vehicle have the highest risk of injury.

29. (B) The motionless 2-year-old should be checked first for airway status and breathing. Next you should check the 10-year-old since her airway may also be in jeopardy, perhaps from a crushed larynx. The 34-year-old female can then be assessed for ABCs and internal hemorrhage.

30. (D) You must first open the child's airway. The next action would be to give four quick breaths. If at this point there is no response, triage procedure dictates that the patient who has only a slight chance of survival must not consume the energy that may save another patient's life. If a back-up system were closer, perhaps CPR would be started.

31. (B) A flail chest is defined as more than one rib fractured in more than one place.

32. (D) At this point in her pregnancy, the sudden onset of bleeding without pain is most likely caused by placenta previa. Pain would be expected with active labor, or ruptured uterus. An ectopic pregnancy ruptures at a much earlier stage.

33. (D) Oxygen should be started and antishock trousers should be in place so that they can be inflated if needed, without having to apply the suit en route. (Use of the antishock garment is controversial; check your local protocols.) An IV of normal saline should be initiated.

34. (A) The first priority is to open and maintain patency of the airway. Snoring respirations indicate an occlusion of the airway, which needs immediate attention. Immobilization of the C-spine is accomplished while simultaneously opening the airway. Intubation with in-line stabilization may be indicated as a later priority. Control of bleeding, although important, is also not the first priority.

35. (B) Decerebrate posturing is described as extension. Decorticate posturing, or flexion, is flexing of the arms at the elbow and straightening of the legs. Decerebrate posturing indicates a somewhat more serious injury to the brain stem than decorticate posturing. Tetany is characterized by intermittent spasms of the extremities caused by changes in the pH and extracellular calcium.

36. (A) Increased intracranial pressure is evidenced by an increase in blood pressure due to edema of the brain, causing compromise of arterial perfusion. A fall in blood pressure suggests a hypovolemic state. Bradycardia is a vagal reflex resulting from compression of the brain. Abnormal respiratory patterns occur with increased pressure on the brain stem, and pupillary changes occur as a result of pressure on the third nerve.

37. (B) To avoid damage to the mucosa, suction is applied only while removing the catheter. Suction should never be applied for more than 10 seconds at a time, and the patient should be well-oxygenated between suctioning attempts.

38. (D) Despite the history of emphysema, this patient obviously requires increased delivery of oxygen as evidenced by cyanosis. Be prepared to assist ventilations if the patient's respiratory drive is diminished by the administration of oxygen. Intubation is premature at this point but may be required if the patient's condition deteriorates. Epinephrine is not indicated in the management of emphysema.

39. (C) Antacids are an alkaline substance, and taken in large quantities can produce a metabolic alkalosis. Some antacids are also high in sodium content, which may lead to fluid retention.

40. (B) The usual dosage of nitroglycerine is 0.4 mg (1/150 grains) sublingually every 5 minutes, up to three tablets within 15 minutes. If the systolic blood pressure falls below 100 mm Hg or a drop of 30 mm Hg or greater occurs, withhold any subsequent dose until blood pressure stabilizes.

41. (A) Atropine is contraindicated in the presence of glaucoma. Atropine causes the pupils to dilate, preventing the outflow of aqueous humor and thereby causing increased intraocular pressure. It may, however, be given if required by the patient's clinical condition.

42. (C) Using ABC criteria, the patient has a patent airway but difficulty breathing. Sealing the wound should improve the patient's condition and is therefore the first priority. It will prevent air from rushing into the chest cavity, increasing the size of the pneumothorax. A volume expander IV, spinal immobilization, and cardiac monitor are all appropriate following airway management.

43. (D) Distended neck veins, diminished or absent breath sounds, and hypoxia are all signs of tension pneumothorax. Abdominal pain is not a sign of tension pneumothorax, and the tracheal shift, when observable, is to the unaffected side.

44. (A) The occlusive dressing should be opened when the patient exhales. This may result in an immediate release of pressure and therefore prevent additional complications.

45. (A) A needle thoracostomy may relieve a tension pneumothorax. A tension pneumothorax is considered a life-threatening emergency. As the pneumothorax expands, the lung collapses on the affected side, and if this condition continues without intervention, pressure is exerted on the vital structures of the mediastinum. The patient develops increasing dyspnea and decreased cardiac output due to decreased venous return and pressure against the heart itself.

46. (D) Inserting the needle at the second intercostal space, midclavicular line on the affected side allows air to escape and does not risk injury to vital thoracic structures.

47. (D) This patient should be managed in the same way as other trauma patients; therefore, he should be immobilized. The path of the bullet inside the body is unpredictable, and thus the bullet may have caused a vertebral fracture. A spinal cord injury could have resulted from the fall to the ground as well.

48. (C) Mr. Jones has most likely received a multitude of severe injuries. Shock is a potential, and he should receive high-concentration oxygen as soon as possible. He can be examined for skin color changes in the mouth or for capillary refilling in the nail beds. Bleeding from a complete amputation will usually be controlled by the retraction and constriction of the blood vessels of the stump. Mr. Jones should receive care to potentially life-threatening problems before attention is given to the amputated limb.

49. (D) Proper care for amputated body parts includes wrapping the part in a sterile dressing, placing it in a plastic bag, and then placing the bag in an ice chest. The tissue should not be in direct contact with the ice. Local protocols vary regarding whether to place a moist saline dressing

over exposed tissue. Consult your physician advisor. Avoid freezing the part (e.g., dry ice). Avulsed teeth may be kept in a warm solution, milk, or in the patient's mouth if not contraindicated by the patient's level of consciousness.

50. (C) The antishock garment can be applied as soon as Mr. Jones has been freed from the wreckage. Inflate both leg compartments and the abdominal compartment. This will help control bleeding and immobilize both leg injuries and the pelvic fracture. A simple pressure dressing is probably all that is needed on the stump.

Bibliography

American Academy of Orthopaedic Surgeons. **Emergency Care and Transportation of the Sick and Injured**. 5th ed. Chicago: A.A.O.S., 1992.

American Heart Association. **Textbook of Advanced Cardiac Life Support**. 2nd ed. Dallas: American Heart Association, 1987.

American Heart Association. **Textbook of Pediatric Advanced Life Support**. Dallas: American Heart Association, 1988.

Bledsoe, Bryan E. **Atlas of Paramedic Skills**. Englewood Cliffs, NJ: Brady/Prentice Hall, 1988.

Bledsoe, Bryan E., Robert S. Porter and Bruce Shale. **Paramedic Emergency Care**. Englewood Cliffs, NJ: Brady/Prentice Hall, 1991.

Bledsoe, Bryan E., Gideon Bosker and Frank J. Papa. **Prehospital Emergency Pharmacology**. 3rd ed. Englewood Cliffs, NJ: Brady/Prentice Hall, 1992.

Campbell, John, M.D. **Basic Trauma Life Support**. Englewood Cliffs, NJ: Brady/Prentice Hall, 1988.

Caroline, Nancy L., M.D. **Ambulance Calls: Review Problems for the Paramedic**. 3rd ed. Boston: Little, Brown and Company, 1991.

Caroline, Nancy L., M.D. **Emergency Care in the Streets**. 4th ed. Boston: Little, Brown and Company, 1991.

Copass, Michael K., et al. **The Paramedic Manual**. 2nd ed. Philadelphia: W.B. Saunders Company, 1987.

Cotton, Sherrie L. **Paramedic Review Guide**. St. Louis: Mosby-Yearbook, Inc., 1989.

Edwards, David P., and Mark Weingartner. **Paramedic Examination Review Manual**. Englewood Cliffs, NJ: Brady/Prentice Hall, 1991.

Gazzaniga, Alan B., M.D., et al. **Emergency Care: Principles and Practices for the EMT-Paramedic**. 2nd ed. Reston, VA: Reston Publishing Company, Inc., a Prentice Hall Company, 1982.

Grant, Harvey D., Robert H. Murray, Jr. and J. David Bergeron. **Emergency Care**. 5th ed. Englewood Cliffs, NJ: Brady/Prentice Hall, 1990.

Greenwald, Jonathan. **The Paramedic Manual**. Englewood, CO: Morton Publishing Company, 1988.

Hafen, Brent Q., and Keith J. Karren. **Prehospital Emergency Care & Crisis Intervention**. 3rd ed. Englewood, CO: Morton Publishing Company, 1990.

Phillips, Charles, M.D. **Paramedic Skills Manual**. Bowie, MD: Robert J. Brady Co., a Prentice Hall Company, 1980.

Pre-Hospital Trauma Life Support Committee of the National Association of Emergency Medical Technicians in Cooperation with the Committee on Trauma of the American College of Surgeons, **Pre-Hospital Trauma Life Support**. Akron, OH, Educational Direction, Inc., 1986.

Ptacnik, Donald J. **Review Manual for the EMT-Intermediate**. 3rd ed. Los Altos, CA: National Nursing Review, Inc., 1990.

Ptacnik, Donald J. **The EMT Review Manual: Self-Assessment Practice Tests**. 3rd ed. Los Altos, CA: National Nursing Review, Inc., 1990.

Simon, Joseph E. **Pediatric Life Support Manual**. St. Louis: Mosby-Yearbook, Inc., 1988.

Stewart, Charles, M.D., and Carol P. Stewart. **Emergency Medical Technician Paramedic Examination Review**. New York: Medical Examination Publishing Company, 1989.

U.S. Department of Transportation. **Emergency Medical Technician–Paramedic: National Standard Curriculum**. Washington, DC: U.S. Department of Transportation, National Highway Traffic Safety Administration, 1985.

Walraven, Gail. **Basic Arrhythmias**. 3rd ed. Englewood Cliffs, NJ: Brady/Prentice Hall, 1991.

Walraven, Gail, and Miles Julihn. **Paramedic Review Guide**. 3rd ed. Englewood Cliffs, NJ: Brady/Prentice Hall, 1991.

Wiegel, Al, James Atkins and James Taylor. **Automated Defibrillation**. Englewood, CO: Morton Publishing Company, 1988.